Live Your Life with COPD – 52 Weeks of Health, Happiness and Hope

Live Your Life with COPD *contains all the pearls of wisdom from a practicing clinician who has taken care of a large number of COPD patients, and could have only been written by someone who has fought in the trenches. [This book] belongs in every person's home that has a chronic lung disease.*
   – Larry Westby, MS, RRT

Jane has done a wonderful job of combining Jo-Von's editorials with her own knowledge, experience and teachings to compile this informative, easy-to-follow guide to understanding and learning to live with COPD. She truly is dedicated to helping us live better lives with this disease. Thanks, Jane for all your hard work, your love and caring.
   – Peg Auwerda, COPD and Pulmonary Rehab patient

This book will help me deal with my disease day-by-day, week-by-week, and month-by-month. I found it to be absolutely uplifting and empowering because of the knowledge and courage it provided me. I'll be keeping it on my nightstand always.
   – Neva Maynor, person with COPD /
   Alpha-1 Antitrypsin Deficiency

Live Your Life with COPD: 52 Weeks of Health Happiness and Hope *combines the editorials of famed COPD advocate and 'thriver', the late Jo-Von Tucker, with Jane's unique writing style and expertise in COPD* *education. The final product is a wonderful book that allows the reader to get a perspective they can relate to that isn't sterile and fact-driven, like much of the COPD information out there. A nice touch in this book is the 52-week format used, allowing readers to contemplate and apply principles that will help them achieve 'Health, Happiness, and Hope'!*

– Craig Ammerall, RRT-CPFT
Author of *Breathwish: A Scriptural Guide to Smoking Cessation and Understanding COPD*

A must read for anyone struggling to live with COPD. Jane shows us how to keep quality in our lives, rather than letting the disease overwhelm and over power us.

– Margo, COPD patient

The combination of JoVon Tucker's classic editorials on COPD and information from Jane Martin's latest Internet blogs and postings prove to be a wonderful way to learn how to live with respiratory problems. If you have COPD or are a loved one or health professional caring for those who do, you will benefit from reading **Live Your Life with COPD: 52 Weeks of Health, Happiness and Hope.**

– Celeste Belyea RRT RN AE-C
The Pulmonary Paper

It has been said that knowledge is power. Jane has used her knowledge as a respiratory therapist along with Jo-Von's experience as a COPD patient to help you gain that power. This book offers you, the reader, information to understand what is happening to your body and support for how to maintain the very best quality of life while slowing the progression of your disease.

– Ted Jones, a survivor with COPD

As a person with very severe COPD I highly recommend this book. As I read through it, I realize that others really do understand what I am dealing with. Depression, guilt, anger, good days-bad days, loss of quality of life and activities are so much a part of life with COPD. It can be overwhelming and frustrating and yes, very scary. Jane helps us understand what is going on and how to help ourselves as much as possible.

    – Phil H., COPD patient

Live Your Life with COPD

52 Weeks of Health, Happiness and Hope

Based on the editorials of Jo-Von Tucker

Jane M. Martin, BA, LRT, CRT

ISBN 0-7414-6435-7

Printed in the United States of America

Published March 2011

INFINITY PUBLISHING
1094 New DeHaven Street, Suite 100
West Conshohocken, PA 19428-2713
Toll-free (877) BUY BOOK
Local Phone (610) 941-9999
Fax (610) 941-9959
Info@buybooksontheweb.com
www.buybooksontheweb.com

This book is dedicated to the people with Chronic Obstructive Pulmonary Disease (COPD):

Those to whom I've listened and those who've heard me as I've taught, nodding as the light went on and saying, "Thank you. I finally understand this."

You humble me.
You honor me.
You are my teachers.
You are my inspiration.

Medical Disclaimer

This book is not intended as medical advice, nor to take the place of an authorized medical professional. You, the reader, are encouraged to discuss the information in this book with your personal physician or other qualified respiratory care professional so together, you can determine the best treatment and care for your individual situation.

Contents – Calendar Method

Contents – Content Method

The Basics

Relationships

Day-to-Day Living

Emotional Issues and Coping

Living and Dying with COPD

Just for Fun

Acknowledgments

I am grateful to Jo-Von Tucker, for having not only the insight to look inward and the skill to write about emotions in life with COPD, but the courage to put it out there. I am thankful to Dr. Austin "Bill" Kutscher for trusting me with Jo-Von's editorials and affirming their importance; and to Tracy Rolsten for her support in making sure her mother's words live on.

My heartfelt appreciation goes to all the members of my Breathing Better Living Well Team: To my right hand, Eileen, for reading the material early on and assuring me it had to be shared; for ably holding the BBLW fort as I wrote, and for so thoughtfully and meticulously researching many of the excellent resources found in "Your Turn." My thanks goes to Peg, Dee, Neva, and Darrell, my sounding boards and the true COPD experts because they live it every day, and to Steve, for giving us Hope and being my friend. I thank the BBLW RT's, Craig, Larry, and Sandy for understanding the power of online information and support and for standing with me in understanding the unique art, science and passion of respiratory care.

I am indebted to Dr. Robert "Sandy" Sandhaus, Dr. Frank Adams, Dr. Vijai Sharma, Helen Sorenson, RRT, and Larry Westby, RRT for contributing their medical expertise and checking over chapters; to Richard Martin for granting permission to print his piece on airway clearance, to Peg Auwerda for sharing her story about massage, to Josie for telling me stories of her adventures, and to Travis Randolph for his support.

My gratitude goes to LinDee Rochelle for her professionalism as my editor, her patience as my author advocate, and her empathy as a fellow author who understands all too well that there are never enough hours in a day. Thank you to Bob Goodman at Silvercat for transforming my manuscript into this lovely book; to Chris Master, for his artistry in designing the cover and for putting up with my (almost) never-ending tweaks; and to my son, Harrison Martin, for drawing a picture of the lungs.

I thank my writer friends who were there when I needed them with comments and suggestions – both gentle and not. I appreciate their generosity in showing me the consideration only fellow writers can, but most of all for asking perfect questions, then patiently waiting with me through that sometimes terrifying silence until I found the answers myself.

Boundless appreciation is owed to my mother for her unflagging support of my work and, without fail, listening to me babble on every Monday morning; to my children, Corinne and Harrison, for reminding me that when it comes right down to it, I'm just me; and to my amazing husband, Marvin, for taking care of a thousand everyday things with never a complaint, and giving me the space to write. But most of all, for loving me as I am, and always – and forever – being there.

Finally, I thank my patients. You are the reason I love what I do. You teach me something every single day. You lift me up.

Introduction

A Story of Two Women

I didn't choose to write this book. It chose me.

When I was writing my first book in 1999, I heard about a yet-to-be published book, *Courage and Information for Life with Chronic Obstructive Lung Disease.* I was excited to learn of this new book about COPD – especially one written by a patient – a lady named Jo-Von Tucker. As soon as it was available for sale I bought it.

As I read it I was struck by Jo-Von's honesty in telling what it was like for her to fight the day-to-day battle for health and breath. The emotional issues in life with COPD can be brutal. In her writing Jo-Von talk about them, courageously baring herself to readers, revealing her fears, her demons, her failings, her triumphs – her hopes.

She wrote about the very issues – the emotional struggles – I'd seen in my own patients. On the road they traveled, sometimes my patients would stumble and fall; at times it was as if they were swallowed by a sinkhole. More often than not, though, they'd pick themselves up and march on, even stronger than before. But every time, every single time – by just being assured they were not alone – they were inspired.

I, myself, don't have COPD, but from my experiences working with people (at that time it had been for nearly 20 years) I knew more than anything that this information about life with COPD, must come to light. That's why I decided to write my first book; so folks with COPD who were doing well, those who'd faced the issues and conquered them, could help others. And thanks to Jo-Von I'd found even more insight.

I was in awe of this woman, Jo-Von Tucker, who had not only beaten the odds to live on – and live well – with COPD but had written a comprehensive guide to living with COPD. After all, she was a successful business-woman, who, at age 52 was diagnosed with COPD and told she had two to five years to live. Undaunted, she marched on to become a well-known advocate for people with COPD, a support group leader, speaker and writer.

So, with a leap of faith I contacted her through email, not sure if she'd open the note in the first place, give me another thought if she did, let alone write back. But she did. We soon became friends and supported each other in both our writing and in the often challenging process of publishing. When others were writing about things like medications and nutrition, yes, we were writing about that – but so much more. We wrote about what was in the hearts and minds of people with COPD. Jo-Von and I were kindred spirits in that regard; pretty much the only ones back then writing about the emotional issues associated with COPD.

Jo-Von added me to the mailing list for her Cape Cod Support Group newsletter. I looked forward each month to seeing what was going on with her group because I, too, ran a support group in my hometown. But without a doubt, the first piece I'd look for was her editorial. So often I'd think, "Boy, she hit the nail on the head with this one! Real people feel this way, but they just don't talk about it. And here she is, putting it down on paper."

Our friendship grew. Jo-Von introduced me by phone to a colleague of hers, Dr. Austin "Bill" Kutscher who organized COPD symposiums at Columbia University Hospital in New York City. In November of 2003 I finally met both Jo-Von and Bill in person at the first national COPD Coalition Conference in Arlington, Virginia. I first came upon Jo-Von who was sitting in a wheel chair in front of her presentation in the poster room. I met Bill later that night. He was a wiry man in his eighties; not as tall as I, but with an energy and intensity that was ferocious. I was honored to be in their company and it struck me then – there was so much for me to learn.

Barely a month later I was shocked and saddened to learn that Jo-Von passed away unexpectedly from complications following surgery. In corresponding with her over three years through email, I'd always looked forward to meeting her someday but also to working with her. That latter hope, of course, was now gone. Or, was it?

The following June I was invited to speak at a COPD symposium organized by Bill at Columbia University Medical Center in New York City. The focus was "Volunteerism in COPD." Bill had asked me to present two papers; one I'd written, and the other written by Jo-Von, one she had planned to present. At the close of the first day of the event, Bill handed me a stack of papers held together by a rubber band.

"Jane, these are Jo-Von's editorials. You should have them."

"Um…okay…thank-you," I answered, not really understanding what he meant by giving them to me, nor knowing what he wanted me to do with them.

That night in my hotel room, I read them, one after the other, spreading them out on my bed. I was overcome again by the wisdom in those forty-some editorials within 150 pages of her writings. It was a joy to see Jo-Von's words, the entire collection here in front of me – these open, positive, hopeful expressions of a wise woman. It was a delight to read with a fresh eye her experiences, her advice, her insight, her questions, as she shared her mind and heart and spirit – and doing it with gusto and that no-nonsense Texas / Manhattan style. I knew that night – somehow this work must be shared so Jo-Von's legacy could live on.

The next day at the symposium I approached Bill. "I read the editorials."

His piercing eyes met mine. "Yes."

I thought, "Jane, you've got an awful lot of nerve, but you have to say what you believe. I came right out with it. "They should be in a book."

He smiled. "I was hoping you'd say that. And you're the one to do it."

I was stunned; first, by Bill's trust in me, and a moment later, with the weight of this responsibility. That was 2004. Now, six years later, I've completed the job. I've done what Bill asked me to do and what I'm sure Jo-Von, also, would have wanted. I regret I never had the honor to work with my friend directly, but in working with her editorials – her thoughts, her words – I finally did. It's been a joy and an honor. Here and now, I humbly pick up the torch I was given, and together, we go on.

This was the last editorial written by Jo-Von Tucker. It appeared in the November 2003 issue of the Cape Cod Support Group Newsletter, just weeks before her death. In it, Jo-Von tells her story.

November 2003
A Patient's Perspective on Living with COPD
by Jo-Von Tucker

On October 16, I traveled to Sturbridge, Mass. to give a speech for the American Lung Association at the Massachusetts Society for Respiratory Care Conference. I reprinted this speech for this issue of our Newsletter. Bear in mind that the audience for the talk was several hundred respiratory therapists and pulmonary medical professionals. I wanted to give them a very personal and insightful look into the lives of their patients.

Fourteen years ago I walked out of a lung specialist's office at National Jewish Hospital in Denver, Colorado, in a state of shock. I had been diagnosed with something called COPD, which I later discovered stood for Chronic Obstructive Pulmonary Disease. I had absorbed little in the distress of this meeting, but I did come away with the facts that COPD is a chronic illness, incurable, and usually progressive.

With the jolting news that I would have to be on supplemental oxygen for the rest of my life, and that the prognosis for my life was between two and five years, I hauled myself away like a wounded bear. At that time I wanted only to get back home to my apartment in New York City, and to be given some time to think about this devastating turn of events. I took the next plane back to Manhattan, after pleading with American Airlines officials to bend the rules and supply me with oxygen on the flight home.

Back home I tried to hide the portable oxygen unit from the doorman of my building, and then from the elevator operators in the lobby. I don't know why I was seized with the need to conceal the oxygen equipment...after all, I wore a nasal cannula that was clearly in sight. Maybe it's because I just didn't have the emotional strength to explain the sudden appearance in my life of oxygen paraphernalia.

By this time, I had deliberately chosen life over death; survival over giving in to a disease that I sensed could engulf me quickly. After several weeks of isolation and grief, as I emerged from shock, I began to need answers...some of which may have been given to me in Denver, but managed to disappear in the dark cloud of the reality that surrounded me. I went to large bookstores in Manhattan. I haunted the public library looking for information about COPD, anything that could help me better understand it – and fight it. I searched the Internet. I researched health newsletter, from The Mayo Clinic to a couple of grass roots cyber organizations.

Precious little information was available. So I pieced together all that I could find and studied like I was preparing for a college term exam. I know I am a fighter. But I also know that I handle situations much better if I know exactly what I am dealing with. So I attempted to fill in the blanks. Years later, from experience and my own research, I was able to write my book about COPD, providing help and encouragement for other people who were facing the same diagnosis.

Why am I telling you all of this? Because the lack of information I encountered about COPD fourteen years ago still exists to some extent.

I'm attempting to bring to this audience, most of whom are medical professionals, a little perspective about COPD – perspective from the patient's life. In spite of the education and special knowledge that you may have received, you truly cannot know how we, the COPD patients, feel unless you have walked a bit in our shoes.

Of course you know the physiological symptoms of COPD...extreme shortness of breath, frequent exacerbations of lung infection, lack of tolerance for exercise, weakness and fatigue. But did you also know that we suffer from periodic bouts of depression? There are many reasons for this, including grieving for the things we can no longer do because of our physical limitations. Plus, we are dealing with a hidden disease – one that is not overtly obvious to people around us unless we happen to be sporting a nasal cannula.

COPD can lead to isolation. People with lung disease may cut themselves off, deliberately or not, from their families, close friends, co-workers and neighbors, because it takes too much effort to get out of bed and get dressed for socializing. Also because it takes too much of our breath and scarce energy to be with people. And because we must try to protect ourselves from common colds and viruses, which can, literally bring us down.

Isolation, in turn, leads to more depression. Depression paralyzes us with an inability to move...to exercise, which we must do to stay as conditioned as possible; to remain vital within our own families and communities. The BIG killer related to COPD may not be the frequent bouts of pneumonia we are susceptible to. It may simply be the loss of quality of life, and companionship. I've seen it happen far too often.

I would not wish this catastrophic illness on anyone. But if you'd care to walk in our shoes for a moment, imagine that you can no longer take a walk on a beach because the sand pulls at your feet like quicksand as it sucks away any strength you have. You cannot lift up your grandchildren for a welcoming hug. You find it very difficult to shop for your own groceries. You probably won't accept social invitations knowing the price you will pay for the effort to go out. You have difficulty even walking across a room. That's what it feels like.

We have one solace available to us, and that is participation in a COPD support group. It provides us with a place we can go to be with others who understand exactly how we feel. Support groups can provide excellent information about the disease, along with coping mechanisms to help us in our battle. We don't feel stared at with our oxygen equipment. And we are able to see other COPD patients, some of whom are much worse than we are, and some who are managing quite well. Both extremes inspire us.

Every COPD person should have access to a vital and active support group. You can best help your patients by encouraging them to visit a group, or to receive a newsletter about the group. If you aren't aware of a local Better Breathers Club in your area, ask The American Lung Association. They'll know where these groups are. In fact, they help many of them by sponsoring them, limited financially and whole-heartedly emotionally.

In closing, let me say that all is not gloom and doom for COPDers. Each new day that dawns may be the one in which research scientists find the answer to generating new lung tissue. It may be the day that another COPD patient is able to achieve stability, slowing or halting the downward spiral of deterioration. It might be the day when we are able to reach out to lung patients to let them know that, with careful management of their illness, they may be able to hold on to a greater degree of that quality of life.

I hope it hasn't been too painful for you to walk temporarily in my shoes. I deeply appreciate your interest, your attention, and your professional expertise.

Underneath the text of her speech Jo-Von shared this quote:

Man's main concern is not to gain pleasure or to avoid pain but rather to see a meaning in his life. That is why man is even ready to suffer, on the condition, to be sure, that his suffering has a meaning.
                                                – Viktor Frankl

How to Get the Most out of This Book

Live Your Life with COPD: 52 Weeks of Health, Happiness and Hope is organized as a perpetual calendar with 52 chapters, one for each week of the year. Some chapters focus on seasonal events or specific concerns relevant to that time of year.

People with COPD often feel overwhelmed with all there is to learn when it comes to managing this disease: Medications, breathing techniques, nutrition, pacing, oxygen, not to mention the wide array of emotional issues. The one chapter per week structure in *Live Your Life* was designed to give you, the reader, one aspect of COPD to focus on per week, allowing you time to learn the subject.

But as solid as this information may be, reading is still passive. This is why at the end of each chapter you'll find "Your Turn," which includes key points, thoughtful questions, suggested tasks and goals, as well as additional resources. This will help you think about how the topic relates to you, and put solutions into practice. (Every effort was made for the resources in "Your Turn" to include on line resources for computer users as well as those in hard copy and phone numbers for readers who do not go online. If you are unable to connect with any Internet resource listed in this book, type the name of the resource into a search engine, such as Google or Yahoo, and a current link to that resource should appear.)

At the end of some chapters there is a "Bonus Box." In the Bonus Box you'll discover something extra; additional information or inspiration having to do with that chapter.

By all means, if this is your copy of *Live Your Life with COPD*, I wholeheartedly encourage you to write your own notes and thoughts in the book itself. If you've borrowed this copy from a friend or library, keep a notebook with it so you, too, can participate in "Your Turn."

There are two different ways to use this book.

1. Calendar Method

If you choose the calendar method, when you open this book for the first time, start in on that week of the year. Let's say you're ready to start reading and it happens to be the fourth week in April. In that case you would start with the chapter "April – Week 4 – Coping with Stress." From there you can go right on through to the end of the book, then continue on with "January – Week 1" until you finish with "April – Week 3 –Nutrition."

2. Content Method

If you prefer learning first about the Basics of living with COPD, such as lung function, medications, nutrition, exercise, etc., see the alternate Table of Contents – Content Method. This organizes chapters by categories and topics.

If you wish to sit down and read right through the book at your own pace, of course you may do that! Or, if you feel like skipping around to chapters that interest you at the moment, feel free. If you choose to do this, however, leave a checkmark in the Table of Contents for chapters you've covered. 52 chapters is a lot to keep track of and I wouldn't want you to miss anything!

Welcome to *Live Your Life with COPD – 52 Weeks of Health, Happiness and Hope,* your guide to living well with COPD. I wish for you the discovery of solid help for better breathing, thoughtful perspectives, joyful inspiration and endless empowerment. Whether you were diagnosed ten years ago, or just yesterday, come along with us now on this journey, a journey of not just weeks – but years – of *Health, Happiness and Hope.*

A Word from the Author

On Teaching and Learning

For thirty years I've had the honor – and the privilege – to teach people with COPD about the many aspects of living with this disease; from their lungs and how they work, to coping with denial and guilt and many topics in between. I've spoken to gatherings as small as five, I've made presentations to groups of several hundred at conferences and educational events, and everything in between.

For me, the reward of teaching is when I look into the faces of my patients or those in the audience and see them nod, see them smile, see them laugh when I offer a bit of humor, see welling eyes as I speak of something life-changing and profound – and then, after the presentation when they come up and say, "Thank you. This makes sense to me now. I finally understand it."

Here, I humbly offer my words – words I've shared with people with COPD and have been told they were helpful – in hopes that they will inform, educate, inspire, and comfort you, as well. I don't claim to know all there is to know about effective pulmonary management with COPD. Far from it. In fact, after working in this field for over thirty years, I discover each day that there is more and more I don't know. And in the six years I've worked with this material, compiling, integrating, and editing, I've continue to learn. So, dear reader, as you make your way through *Live Your Life*; as you take this journey, know I'm learning right along with you.

Credits

This book is based on and inspired by, in large part, the editorials of my friend, the late Jo-Von Tucker. Some chapters are essentially unchanged from the originals. These chapters are credited as JVT. Other chapters originating from her editorials have been updated and / or more significantly edited, and in doing so, I've done my best to be true to her message and her voice. These chapters are credited as JVT/JMM. All chapters originated by Ms. Tucker are written in first person.

Most of the remaining chapters, authored by me, are written in second and third person and credited as JMM.

Chapters provided by respiratory health care professionals and others indicate their original authorship by name and JMM if significantly edited.

What is COPD?

COPD, Chronic Obstructive Pulmonary Disease, is an umbrella term used to describe progressive lung diseases which include emphysema, chronic bronchitis, refractory (irreversible) asthma, and severe bronchiectasis.[1]

Symptoms of COPD:

* Frequent coughing, often producing phlegm
* Shortness of breath while doing everyday activities
* Shortness of breath with the inability to keep up with others your own age
* Wheezing and / or chest tightness

COPD Facts

* It is estimated that 12 million adults in the US have COPD, and another 12 million are undiagnosed or developing COPD.[2]
* COPD is the third leading cause of death in the U.S.[3]
* It is estimated that over 210 million people worldwide have COPD.[3]
* Smoking is the major (but not the only) cause of COPD. Second-hand smoke, occupational dust and chemicals, air pollution, and genetic factors can also cause COPD.

1. COPD Foundation http://www.Copdfoundation.org
2. The National Heart, Lung, and Blood Institute (NHLBI) http://www.nhlbi.nih.gov
3. COPD Foundation http://www.Copdfoundation.org

* COPD is easy to diagnose using spirometry, a brief and easy test in which the patient exhales as much air as possible into a tube.
* While there is currently no cure for COPD, it is mostly preventable and very treatable.

You are at risk for having COPD if:

* You cough on most days
* You bring up phlegm or mucus on most days
* You get out of breath more easily than others your age
* You are 45 years or older
* You are a current smoker or an ex-smoker
* You have history of environmental chemicals, dust, or fumes in the workplace, heavy or long-term contact with secondhand smoke or other lung irritants.

Happy New Year!
[JVT]

The successful man is one who had the chance and took it.
    – Roger Babson

A new year has begun, and with it, another opportunity to take control of our breathing – and our lives – with COPD. We enter a whole new year armed with actions we can take to improve our lung health; to stay active and fit, to follow our physicians' treatment plan as prescribed, to strengthen our commitment to socialize and avoid isolation, and to look at that glass not as half empty, but always half full.

We have much to gain in this, making a New Year's resolution to breathe better. We can achieve a level of stability and remain well from day to day as opposed to helplessly watching our health spin out of control and spiral into steady and swift decline! Stability for COPDers may appear fragile, but it doesn't have to be that way.

We can, and should, devote our energy to maintaining an active role in the management of our health. Side-by-side with our doctors and loved ones, we can be responsible for our health management – whatever is required to help balance our lives in our quest for improved health.

Our doctors can guide us, direct us, and measure our success. Our family members can encourage and inspire us to be faithful with our regular exercise routine, take our medicines and to get the nutrition we need. They can even go along with us to doctor appointments and support group meetings. Our respiratory therapists can help keep us on our toes regarding the proper use of supplemental oxygen and equipment, if it has been prescribed. They can test our oximetry to be sure we are getting the maximum benefit from our O_2 (oxygen). And they will also pretty much know if we are using our oxygen as it has been prescribed for us.

Many people can be of help to us as we fight the good fight against lung disease... **But they can't do it for us!** They can advise, they can cajole (although they shouldn't have to), and they can cheer from the sidelines whenever we've won a major battle with an exacerbation. But they cannot do the exercises for us, they cannot take our medicines for us, and they certainly cannot breathe for us! We are the ones who must be responsible for our accomplishments in health management!

So, you and me, let's make our New Year's Resolution right now, to commit ourselves to whatever it takes to have stability in our lives with COPD – to take control of our breathing – and our lives. We can do it. Now is the time.

Your Turn

Key points, or... If you don't remember anything else, remember this:

- Now is the right time to make a fresh start.
- It is necessary to take responsibility for your own health.
- You **can** be in control of your breathing – and your life.

Ask yourself this:

Have you ever made New Year's resolutions that were just too overwhelming – and then when you couldn't follow through, you became discouraged?

This week:

- Keep it simple. Make a promise to yourself to do at least three of the following to improve your breathing – and stick with it! You can do as many as you want, but it's okay to pick only three. Just start somewhere.
- Tell yourself everyday that you can learn to take control of your breathing.
- Commit to learning just one new thing each week from this book and putting it into practice.
- Learn how your medicines work to open up your lungs. Different breathing medications work in different ways.
- Smile ten times a day.
- Start walking, only one or two minutes at a time if that's all you can do, and add one more minute each day (approved by your doctor, of course).
- Before you go to bed each night, write down something for which you are thankful.
- If you smoke, quit. If you fall down on it, don't be too hard on yourself. Get back up and try again.
- Wear your oxygen as prescribed. Every day.
- Try a new hobby or activity (or get back to something you had been doing but stopped because of your breathing).

Here's more help

- Online information and support for people with COPD, http://www.Breathingbetterlivingwell.com
- *Expert's Guide to Better Breathing* – an excellent booklet about living with COPD. Free of charge. 800-231-6568.

Know Your Numbers –
Pulmonary Function Testing
[JMM]

*Education is learning what you didn't even know
you didn't know.*
– Daniel Boorstin

Have you had your breathing tested and if so, do you know your numbers? You should!

Pulmonary Function Testing is a necessary part of correctly diagnosing COPD and other lung disorders. Your doctor wouldn't diagnose a patient with hypertension (high blood pressure) without taking a blood pressure reading, or diagnose a patient with diabetes without ever testing the blood sugar level. Just the same, if you have trouble breathing, or if you are at risk for COPD (see the quiz at the end of this chapter) you should have a pulmonary function test. Once the results are in, you should know your numbers just as people with diabetes, cholesterol, and high blood pressure know theirs.

There are two levels of pulmonary function testing: Complete Pulmonary Function, and Pulmonary Function Screen or Spirometry (spy-ráh-meh-tree). A complete pulmonary function test takes about an hour. It tests for flow (how the air moves through your bronchial tubes or airways), volume (how much air your lungs hold), resistance (how elastic or how stiff your lungs are), and diffusion (how well the oxygen moves from your lungs into your bloodstream). A pulmonary function screen, or spirometry, measures only the flow and volume of air

41

moving in and out of your lungs. Spirometry is the short, quick version of a complete pulmonary function test and can usually determine whether or not you have COPD.

The results of a spirometry test can provide information to you and your doctor about whether or not your lungs are functioning normally. If the test results are not normal, it most likely will determine whether the problem with your lungs is obstructive (trouble getting the air out, as in COPD) or restrictive (trouble getting the air in). Once your doctor has the results of your spirometry, he or she may order more tests – maybe a Pulmonary Function Complete – to see more specifically what the problem is.

Your testing begins with determining what your *normal predicted* lung function should be. The technician or therapist conducting the test will ask questions such as, "What is your age, your gender, your height, your race?" The pulmonary function machine knows what the numbers should be for a person with your characteristics and perfectly healthy lungs. Next, you perform the test and your actual results are compared to the normal predicted.

Your final test result is called *percent of normal predicted*. For example, if a person with perfect lungs who is your age, your height, your gender, and your race, would normally blow out two liters of air on a certain maneuver and your best effort results in exhaling one liter, the result of that portion of the test would be 50% of normal predicted. Test results of a pulmonary function screen or spirometry, as well as a complete pulmonary function, will give your doctor and you many different numbers, each one pointing to your percent of normal predicted.

One key indicator of COPD is a decrease in FEV_1. This is the Forced Expiratory Volume that you are able to breathe out in the first second of a long exhalation. Remember, when you have COPD, you have trouble getting your air *out*. If you have COPD you should know your FEV_1 number and perform spirometry regularly to watch for a decline in lung function.

Although your lung function numbers (whether you have lung disease or not) go down with age, the goal is to maintain your numbers as much as possible and slow down or arrest your progression of COPD. Although your FEV_1 might vary a bit from year to year, if you have COPD, you cannot expect it to go up, even if you have an overall improvement in your ability to function in daily activities.

How do you know if you should have spirometry done?

Ask yourself the following questions:

* Are you forty-five years old or older, currently smoke cigarettes or have smoked in the past?
* Are you forty-five years old or older and have a history of breathing irritants in your home environment or work place?
* Did you have recurring pneumonia or trouble breathing as a child?
* Do you sometimes have coughing fits or trouble breathing when exerting?
* Do you have frequent bouts of bronchitis?
* Do you cough up mucus or phlegm on most days?
* Does asthma, bronchitis or emphysema run in your family?
* Do you become short of breath and have trouble keeping up with others your age?

If you can answer yes to any of these questions, ask your doctor if you can be tested with spirometry.

Your Turn

Key points, or … If you don't remember anything else from this chapter, remember this:

- If you have trouble breathing, you should have your lung function tested.
- If you are diagnosed with COPD, you should know your FEV_1 and what that means for you.

Ask yourself this:

- When is the last time you had spirometry?
- What is your FEV_1?

This week:

- Write yourself a note to ask the doctor at your next checkup if you should have spirometry to check on the stability (or progression) of your COPD.
- If you've had a lung function test and don't know your FEV_1, call the facility where you had the test and ask for a copy.

Here's more help

- COPD Foundation
  http://www.copdfoundation.org/
- COPD Information line phone number
  866-316-COPD (2673)

Your Relationship with Your Doctor
[JVT/JMM]

It takes as much energy to wish as it does to plan.
– Eleanor Roosevelt

Aside from the close relationships with your spouse and family members, the next most important person in your life, if you are a lung patient, is your doctor. So, how is your relationship with your primary care physician and your pulmonary specialist? Do you come away from checkups with your questions answered, satisfied with your medical treatment program, and feeling empowered in dealing with your situation? If not, perhaps you should take a good look at the relationship between you and your doctor. As you do, you'll have to take a hard look at your own involvement, as much as you do at his or her guidance.

As patients, we have a role to play in the management of our disease. And we cannot fulfill that role if we are intimidated by the authority of physicians. Living day after day with a chronic disease can, naturally, cause us to feel vulnerable, especially if we have little knowledge of medicine. As patients, we have to work at asserting ourselves and maintaining self-confidence in interactions with our doctors. We should have an equal role of responsibility – letting the doctor know that we expect respect and consideration just as we give the same in return to him or her.

We should tell our doctors, up front, that we'll do our best to follow the prescribed treatment plan. Yet, we must also inform them that we may have many questions in order to understand fully what is going on inside our lungs, what is required of us, and what the desired results should be.

A good physician should welcome your informed approach; and a good doctor knows that the more we know about our disease, the better we can manage it and hold onto as much quality of life as possible. If your doctor says that you "ask too many questions," you may need to think about finding a new doctor – one who isn't threatened by questions, but accepts you as a patient eager to know what's going on. Our doctors should accept us as equal partners in the treatment of our COPD.

Doctors are busy and keep tight schedules. In order to get as much as we can from each appointment with our doctors and respect their time as well, here are some tips.

Seven Ways to Get the Most Out of Your Next Doctor Appointment

1. Think of your doctor as an equal partner in caring for your health – not someone who has all the answers while you don't know anything.
2. Write your questions in between appointments whenever you think of them. Keep them where you can find them, and bring them to your next appointment.
3. Be organized. Get a folder or notebook to hold your health information: Test results, a list of your current medications, and materials (in brief) that relate to your disease.

4. When you see your doctor, state your concerns clearly, taking just one to two minutes. You can say a lot in that time if you're organized. Tell him or her about changes in your breathing and your overall health, since your last appointment.
5. Know what medications you're taking, their names, and what they're supposed to do for you. If you don't know – or if you aren't sure you're using your inhaled medicines properly – ask!
6. Be honest. If you're still smoking and / or taking more of your inhalers than prescribed, your doctor must know.
7. Respect your doctor's time. Health care providers see a different patient every fifteen to thirty minutes all day long, and most of them are doing the very best they can to help you. Do your part to help them too.

Your Turn

Key points, or … If you don't remember anything else from this chapter, remember this:

- You and your doctor should be partners in managing your COPD.
- The more informed you are, the better you will be able to help yourself.
- Keep your health information together in a folder or notebook along with questions for your next appointment.

Ask yourself this:
- Does your doctor listen to what you're trying to say?

- Do you feel comfortable asking your doctor questions? As a respiratory therapist I'm often approached by patients who begin with, "I know this is a stupid question, but..." Please, don't worry about that. The only stupid question is the one you don't ask.

This week:

Make a list of questions about

- Your lung function numbers and your level of disease
- Your treatment program
- If you ask the hard questions, you must be ready to take the hard answers.

Here's more help:

- *The Savvy Patient's Toolkit,* by Margo Corbett.
- *The Savvy Patient: How to Get the Best Health Care,* by Mark Pettus.

Following up... How are you doing on your New Year's Resolutions? If you're still on track, good for you! Keep going! If you've fallen down a bit, don't beat yourself up about it. The important thing is to do *something* to help yourself breathe better. Don't give up! You can do it!

Portions of this chapter excerpted from the article "Get the Most Out of Your Doctor Visit: 7 Things you Need to Know," written by Jane M. Martin, BA, LRT, CRT and published on COPDConnection. com. Copyright 2008 HealthCentral. All rights reserved. http://www. healthcentral.com/copd/c/19257/25200/visit-7

Defying the Laws of Gravity – or Holding on to Stability
[JVT]

You gotta do what you gotta do.
– Sylvester Stallone

My number one commitment – my most important job – is to maintain stability of my disease. Except for a few exacerbations (periods of worsened symptoms, usually due to respiratory infection), over the past fourteen years or so I've maintained a relatively stable condition. I've managed to avoid that slippery slope, the steady downward spiral that can happen to people with COPD. My FEV_1 (Forced Expiratory Volume in the first second of exhalation, a major indicator of severity of COPD) has, until recently, remained mostly the same, with small amounts of decline noted on spirometry (lung function) tests.

Staying stable takes a lot of commitment – to my treatment program, and to staying as conditioned and active as I possibly can. The most difficult part of the search for stability, for me, has been getting enough rest. Working full time, coordinating a breathing support group, writing, editing, and publishing our monthly newsletter, keeping up with the volunteer work for the Emphysema/COPD Composite Program, and serving on the Board of NHOPA (National Home Oxygen Patients' Association), leaves me little time for resting and allowing my body to heal.

That's why the slippery slope of stability seems to me like defying the laws of gravity! Like a skilled trapeze artist from Cirque du Soleil, I've been able to ward off most lung infections, keeping my state of stability in the air at least temporarily, from one stretch to the next.

But like all good things, I suppose that combination of maneuverability and luck had to come to an end sometime. Kerplop! was the sound I seemed to hear as Dr. Mohr reported the latest results of my spirometry test. Gravity – 1, Jo-Von – 0. My lung function numbers had slipped precariously from 60% to about 45% within a short period of time.

Why? Probably several factors: My age, exhaustion, a general de-conditioning that has occurred since I was sick and hospitalized for a couple of weeks with colitis last fall. All combined, a deadly mix that has definitely pulled me down to earth!

I share my personal experience only because I don't want to see it happen to you! We all work to hang on to our stability. I want my example to help you realize your own vulnerability, so you can take steps to preserve the quality of life you've established.

Why is this stability so important? Because once lost, it is extremely difficult to rebuild. Stamina and energy can be improved with the proper steps of management and treatment; but we must remember that our lungs do not regenerate. New replacement tissue will not grow. New functioning alveoli (air sacs in your lungs) will not appear – at least not yet, as scientists continue to work on it. You will naturally lose a tiny bit with time, even if you are successful at holding the disease at bay. Therefore, stability is precious! It is worth expending the effort to hold on to the highest level of COPD possible.

Below is what works for me. I'm passing these suggestions along with hopes that you can hold on to maximum stability as you fight your own battle with this thing we call COPD.

* Listen to your doctor! Understand the treatment program prescribed for you, and follow it. Take your medications exactly as prescribed, including the use of supplemental oxygen.
* Be consistent with your exercise regimen. If you haven't taken a pulmonary rehabilitation course, talk with your doctor about it. If you are a graduate of pulmonary rehab consider taking a refresher course, or at the very least, continue your exercises and physical activities – every day.
* Participate in a breathing support group. Come, listen, talk, question, volunteer, help, learn, share!
* Maintain social contact with the outside world. Do not let this disease rob you of enjoyment and interaction with friends, family, loved ones and neighbors. Isolation leads to depression, and depression can lead to further debilitation.
* Pay attention to nutrition. Feed your body the right foods and nutrients to fuel it in the best way possible. Your body needs protein and a well-balanced diet of fruits, vegetables, meats and dairy products. Take a daily multi-vitamin. Take supplements to put on weight, if necessary.
* Avoid exposure to viruses and cold germs. Wash your hands! Remember to get the flu vaccine when it becomes available in the fall. Ask your doctor about getting a pneumonia vaccine booster if it has been five to seven years since your last shot.

* Pay attention to changes such as a change in the color and / or consistency of your sputum, your regular cough routine, and your usual level of shortness of breath.
* Get enough sleep at night. Sleep disorders are common in people with COPD. Talk with your doctor if you are not sleeping well or do not feel rested in the morning and ask if you should have a sleep study.
* Find the time to give your body the rest that it needs each day. Do not push yourself to exhaustion. If you need an afternoon nap, take one. Listen to your body and do what it tells you to do when it needs a break.

Even if you take all of these pro-active steps and measures, you may still find it hard to attain stability and to maintain it. But it is well worth the effort. Remind yourself that no one can manage your disease for you! It's something you have to do for yourself. Even if you have a loving, caring spouse, there are things about your COPD that only you can know. That's why it's a good idea to keep a journal to write down your notes and thoughts about the ups and downs of your life with this disease. Keep track of good days and bad days, medicines you took, what seemed to help and what didn't. It can serve as a reminder when the situation comes up again.

The search for stability goes on. It may seem to you, too, as though you are trying to defy the laws of gravity. But remember, I've managed to accomplish stability for fourteen years. It took a series of negative circumstances to boot me off that tightrope, but I'm going to get back up there and give it all I've got to make my way to the other side – to stability.

Your Turn

Key points, or . . . If you don't remember anything else from this chapter, remember this:

- It's essential for a person with COPD to maintain stability.
- Follow the treatment plan your doctor – and you – have worked out.
- Know what is normal for you, pay attention when something has changed and take action to stay well.

Ask yourself this:

- Do I cough every day?
- What time of day?
- Do I produce mucous?
- If so, what color is it?
- Is it thick and sticky?

Right now:

Your cough is just one aspect of COPD you should monitor. Start paying attention to your cough and use this chart to jot down the answer / or make a check (√) for a "yes"

	Sun	Mon	Tue	Wed	Thu	Fri	Sat
Do you cough everyday?							
What time of day?							
Do you produce mucous?							
If so, what color is it?							
Is it thick and sticky?							

to these questions every day this week. Ask your doctor about other changes you should watch for, so together, you can fix small problems before they become big ones.

Here's more help:

- Preventing Exacerbations – See chapter September – Week 3
- Your Lung Health http://www.yourlunghealth. org
- American Sleep Apnea Association http://www.sleepapnea.org/ 202-293-3650
- *COPD: The Facts,* by Graeme Currie.
- *The Breathing Disorders Sourcebook,* by Francis Adams, MD.

Reclaiming Your Life through Pulmonary Rehabilitation
[JMM]

The important thing is somehow to begin.
– Henry Moore

One of the biggest issues you, as a person with COPD may be facing is loss – the loss of the ability to do what you used to do, and perhaps the biggest loss of all, control over your breathing, and your life. Pulmonary Rehabilitation can help you regain that strength and control and give you a new start to living well with COPD.

So, what is pulmonary rehab? Below are those six classic questions – Who, what, when, where, why and how – and their answers:

Who should go?

Should I participate in pulmonary rehab? You should discuss this with your doctor if you can answer yes to any of the following questions:

* Do you have COPD and are becoming less physically active?
* Have you had to give up or cut back on activities because of changes brought on by your breathing?
* Are you feeling tired and short of breath (SOB) more often?
* Do you find yourself having frequent bouts of bronchitis, pneumonia, or down with a bad cold

for longer periods of time than other people your age?
* Are you confused about your breathing medications; unsure if they're working or not?
* Do you feel downhearted because of your decline in breathing and activity?
* Do you have COPD with your lung function test showing less than 80% of normal predicted in your FEV_1 or FVC/FEV_1 ratio? (If you have Medicare, it should cover much of the cost of the program. Some other health insurers, or payers, follow Medicare guidelines. As always, check with your health insurance provider for specifics on coverage for you.)

What is it?

Pulmonary rehabilitation is a program of exercise and education especially designed for people with COPD and other chronic lung diseases. In pulmonary rehab you'll gain strength, stamina and flexibility; and learn a lot about your lungs and how to stay as healthy as possible. You'll also find moral support and learn to cope with changes brought on by COPD.

At this point, we should talk about what pulmonary rehab cannot do. Pulmonary rehab cannot cure your lung disease (there is currently no cure for COPD), cannot improve your lung function numbers, or make you feel like you're twenty again!

However, pulmonary rehab can improve your overall physical condition (conditioned muscles require less oxygen) and help you learn to breathe effectively, so you can achieve your maximum potential in spite of your lung disease. It can also give you the control you need to get through episodes of shortness of breath, as well as the confidence to face each day, certain that you know how to take care of your lungs and remain as healthy as possible.

In addition to physical conditioning and effective lung health management, you'll also find ways to cope with lung disease and live your life as fully and happily as possible. Participants in pulmonary rehab often learn the best lessons from each other. After all, they're traveling the same road. People participating in pulmonary rehab often say, "This is the only place I can come where everyone understands what I'm going through."

You might be thinking, "Okay, this sounds all well and good, but I have never been one to exercise. To be honest, I'm kind of scared. What will they make me do in pulmonary rehab?"

While specifics vary, below are the basic components of pulmonary rehab.

Health History

You'll sit down with a nurse and / or a respiratory therapist and talk about your health history. Yes, they will ask if you smoked and if you are still smoking. But, the professionals at pulmonary rehab understand smokers and how hard it is to quit. They're there to help you, not to place blame.

Six-minute walk

You'll walk beside a therapist or nurse while having your oxygen level, heart rate, and blood pressure monitored. The point of the six-minute walk is to see how much distance you can cover in six minutes. Don't worry if you can't walk far. That's why you're there!

Warm up stretches and strengthening

You may work with sticks, resistance bands, and / or light hand weights.

Exercise equipment

Bikes, arm ergometers (peddlers), treadmills, and recumbent steppers are just some of the equipment you'll have the option to use. Remember, the staff at pulmonary rehab specializes in working with people who are short of breath. They'll help you find the best way to exercise in a way that is safe.

Class sessions

You'll learn about proper breathing techniques, medications, nutrition, pacing, conserving energy, relaxation, stress management, developing coping skills, and more.

When would I go?

Pulmonary rehab usually takes place two to three times per week with each session lasting an hour or two. Your time in the program will last from six to twelve weeks, depending on the program. Some offer a continuing maintenance phase in which you may continue after graduation from the monitored program, and come for as long as you want. Many people continue for years in this affordable self-pay phase.

Why should I go to Pulmonary Rehab?

Below are some of the results you can expect if you participate.
 You will:
* Learn about your lung disease and overall health and how to manage it.

* Learn how to breathe more effectively, moving more air with less effort.
* Be more likely to have fewer emergency room visits and hospital admissions due to breathing problems.
* Be in better overall physical condition with more stamina and flexibility.
* Learn coping skills for dealing with your lung disease.
* Experience less anxiety, panic, and feelings of depression about your breathing.
* Have fun while finding friendship and support, knowing you're not alone!

How do I start?

Medicare requires that you have a written referral from your physician, as well as a spirometry or complete pulmonary function done within the last year. If you don't have Medicare, check with your health insurer for specifics of your policy regarding requirements for enrollment and coverage of costs.

Your Turn

Key points, or … If you don't remember anything else from this chapter, remember this:

· Pulmonary Rehabilitation cannot fix your lungs.
· It can help you improve your endurance, strength, and flexibility.
· It can show you how to stay as healthy as possible – even with lung disease – as well as provide encouragement and support.

Ask yourself this:

- Am I ready to give this a try?

This week:

- Ask your doctor if he or she would consider referring you to Pulmonary Rehabilitation.

Here's more help:

- If your doctor or the respiratory staff at your local hospital doesn't know where the nearest pulmonary rehab program is located, contact the AACVPR (American Association of Cardiovascular and Pulmonary Rehabilitation, http://www.aacvpr.org/, 312-321-5146.

Your Relationship with Others
[JVT]

*It is important that the sick person should be
allowed, encouraged, to do all they can. If they
don't, their self worth will vanish.*
– Todd Pierce

Those of us with lung disease may not be aware of the impact of our disease on those around us – especially those closest to us – spouse, friends and family. We often find ourselves more dependent on others as the disease progresses, and as half of a couple, we find we're unable to continue equal sharing in household responsibilities. Those small chores we've always done are no longer within our scope of abilities, due to shortness of breath.

When this happens, we may become angry, hurt, and resentful. Our spouses or family members might also harbor anger and resentment without even knowing it. One person becomes angry at being so dependent and the other is angry about becoming so depended upon. Added to the quotient is guilt; guilt on the patient's part because of feelings of inadequacy for having to rely so heavily on the other party, and guilt on the part of the partner for resenting the added responsibilities.

No matter how physically limited the person with COPD may be, excessive dependency or doting, should be discouraged. It's healthier for people with lung disease to push their restrictions and boundaries as much as safely possible, and frequently they will need encouragement to do so. In this case, "use it or lose it" truly applies.

On the other hand, the wife, husband or partner of the person with COPD needs to be sensitive to indications of frustration and overexertion. These signs may be silently coming from their mate who could be in denial, and showing it, by tackling chores that are clearly beyond their physical abilities. Sometimes patients try to express themselves through non-verbal communication. Perhaps a distressed look signals their partner to just read their mind. The "can't-you-see-I'm-struggling-here?" message is sent. But of course, it truly is unfair to expect someone else to read our thoughts.

This kind of misunderstanding happens with close friends and other family members, as well. When we have visitors or are entertaining at home, patients may try to wait on their guests as they have for many years. We forget that the act of getting up to fix a drink for someone, and then walking across the room to deliver it, will most certainly pull our breath from us. So we may offer to do something for a guest without even thinking about the toll it will take on us. But we should remind ourselves before such a visit that the consequences of overdoing it will not be pleasant for our guests, either. They won't enjoy that glass of wine or iced tea if they have to watch their host gasping for air after getting it for them.

Communication is the key to accomplishing the best understanding and acceptance of our restrictions. And this is true and applicable in all of our relationships; as couples, friends, parents, siblings, or even distant cousins! It is much better to clearly communicate our needs and wishes than it is to risk misunderstood actions and statements.

We have to tell our friends up front about our limitations, rather than trying to hide them. We can do so without dwelling on the issue, simply by honestly stating our situation. Through open discussions with our spouses adjustments can be made as needed about household chores, schedules, and shared responsibilities. Modifications can even make some activities more physically possible than before, such as saying, "Maybe if we just do it this way...Let's try it and see how it works."

It's essential to be open and straightforward about our restrictions. But if we still find that our partner is less understanding than we would like, we should check our own behavior and communication skills. There may be room for improvement there, too. It helps to ask others in our breathing support group, pulmonary rehab class, or on line support group, how they would handle a particular situation. Then we can talk openly and frankly with our partners about expectations on *both* sides.

It is important for COPDers to socialize, and we should be encouraged to do so. Rather than placing all the responsibility on one person for inviting guests over for a chat or a meal, it's better to plan our entertaining objectives together, in advance, with detailed discussions on who will do what. This way our social commitments will become a lot more enjoyable for everyone.

As patients, we have to work hard to maintain self-esteem as we battle our way through the ravages of lung disease. Self-worth becomes elusive when we're faced with the loss of our independence. But when we're successful in communicating as we maintain quality of life – albeit somewhat altered – and when we manage our disease as effectively as possible, we will project an attitude of self-respect. And that is clearly received by those around us – with the same kind of respect sent right back to us. We can then deal effectively with the many emotional issues facing us and be better mates in spite of our disease.

Communication requires work – but our disease doesn't rob us of this ability. By being aware of our relationships, and working to achieve the best understanding, we can do it.

Your Turn

Key points, or … If you don't remember anything else from this chapter, remember this:

- When you have COPD, communication is essential to enjoying a good relationship with others.
- If you have COPD, try to do what you can to contribute to life at home, but recognize your limits.
- Realize that you can't do everything you used to do. Don't be afraid to ask for help. Delegate.
- If you are a caregiver / well spouse of a person with COPD, allow that person do all they can to help around the house. Don't dote on them, but learn their signs of overexertion.

Ask yourself this:

- Do I or my partner have feelings of resentment and guilt in regards to the changes brought on by COPD?

This week:

- If there is tension in your relationships, talk with your spouse, close family members and friends about it. Begin with "I feel…" instead of "you do…" or "you don't…" Using this method is non-accusatory – and no one can ever take it away when you state, "I feel…"

Here's more help:

- Well Spouse Foundation (for family members and other caregivers)
  800-838-0879 http://www.wellspouse.org
- The Spoon Theory http://www.butyoudontlooksick.com

The Need to Love and Be Loved
[JVT/JMM]

*Love is very patient and kind… it is not rude…
it is not easily angered, and it keeps no record of
wrongs… love always protects, always trusts,
always hopes, always perseveres.*
– The Bible: I Corinthians 13:4-8

"With a hose in my nose, a body not even close to what it used to be, and having to fight for breath every day – love and intimacy are the last things on my mind!"

Sound familiar? Having COPD can make it hard to feel lovable. We don't feel well, we don't think we look very good, we can't do what we once could, and we often sense that we're on the outside of a normal, healthy world, looking in.

In spite of our COPD, though, we must hold on to the belief that we are loved – and lovable. This might be one of the most challenging aspects of living with COPD, including that of surviving the physical changes and exacerbations of our disease. But we must be self-affirming, and we must be able to trust in those around us and believe in the love, care, and respect that we receive.

With or without a chronic disease we often tend to be less caring of ourselves than of those around us. Frankly, if we loved our friends and family the way we love ourselves, they'd receive pretty shoddy treatment. At the same time, the less we value ourselves, the harder it is to share loving feelings with others.

It's a basic human need to love and be loved, and if that need is not met, we become stressed. This type of stress can cause us to withdraw from those around us, turn in on ourselves, and nurse our pain. This loneliness can lead to further focus on our ailments, until our lives are ruled by an almost obsessive preoccupation with our body, its functions and malfunctions. Of course, we should be mindful of signs and symptoms of COPD problems, but it is dangerous to be preoccupied with our condition.

Unfortunately, there are those whose own problems keep them from loving us, and in this case we may consider spending less time with them – or avoiding them altogether. We can't fix everyone and everything. We can't solve everyone's problems. We have to love ourselves and we have to take care of ourselves, and this includes steering clear of negativity.

Giving of ourselves – our feelings, hopes, and dreams – despite fears of misunderstanding and rejection, builds the kind of intimacy that relieves the stress of isolation and the agony of disease. Loving others, caring for their needs, surprising them – even delighting them – gives our own life meaning. To give of ourselves in this way requires that we value ourselves and trust that a word or action from us could bring joy to someone.

Even with COPD, we have the power within us to raise someone's spirits, to make his or her day brighter. The healing power of helping others is amazing, and serves us well. We must have the courage to give freely of ourselves, and know in our hearts that the love and trust we accord to others will be returned in kind.

Finally, a word to those of you who have a romantic partner in your life. You may be concerned that your COPD will keep you from expressing yourself intimately with that special person. Know this – even if you're short of breath, you can still engage in sexual intimacy and benefit from the closeness and enjoyment it brings. It may require some changes and adjustments, but you can be intimate.

Hugging, touching and caressing can be satisfying in expressing love with your partner. Talk about it. Feel free to talk, also, with your doctor, nurse, respiratory therapist, or counselor about ways to do this. If they can't help you, they should refer you to someone who can. The resources below have excellent information on intimacy with COPD.

Your Turn

Key points, or... If you don't remember anything else from this chapter, remember this:

- As human beings, we have the need to love and be loved.
- Having COPD can cause us to feel less lovable.
- Even with shortness of breath (SOB), you can be loving and lovable.
- Take care of yourself first.
- Sexual expression comes in many forms and is possible to achieve with COPD, even if you have significant shortness of breath.

Ask yourself this:

- Do I have the support of a loving relationship with someone; a spouse, family member, or close friend who appreciates me? Do I regularly spend time with him or her?

This week:

- Call that special person, send a card or flowers and tell them they mean a lot to you.
- Do something nice for yourself. Go to the barber or salon, buy a new shirt in your favorite color, or indulge in a sweet treat (if safe for your diet, of course!).

Here's more help

- National Jewish Health has excellent, detailed information on relationships and intimacy with COPD. 800-222-5864, http://www.nationaljewish.org

Good Days, Bad Days
[JVT]

This, too, shall pass.
– William Shakespeare

One of the most puzzling aspects in life with COPD is the fact that we have good days, as well as bad days. One day we feel pretty darn good, able to greet the day and do what we want to do. The next day, we find ourselves struggling to breathe with the slightest exertion. Have you heard of a "bad hair" day? This is a "bad air" day – and it's frustrating because it's bad for no obvious reason. It just is – and we all have them.

Worsened shortness of breath is usually the first sign of a bad day. In my own case this is always accompanied by debilitating fatigue, an overwhelming tiredness that makes every little activity a major chore. For our caregivers, spouses and family members, this is a touchy subject that as COPDers, we can't explain. No wonder it's hard for those around us to understand!

What causes those bad days? Why do we feel relatively well one day and the next, suddenly take a turn for the worse? Is the barometric pressure changing? Is it pollen in the air? Is an infection brewing? Did we over exert yesterday? Have we been around someone with a cold or flu virus? Has our diet changed? Are we emotionally upset about something? Is the humidity too high? The list goes on and on. (To learn the early warning signs of a lung infection, see chapter September – Week 3.)

Our choices of ways to deal with those bad days are narrowed considerably by our physical limitations. But deal with them, we must. These are the times we need to call forth all the coping skills we have. Although there are no magic, quick cures for making us feel better, there are ways to get through the bad times.

One of the most important things we can do for ourselves, whether we are fighting an infection or just dealing with a bad day, is to allow extra time for rest. We should always make sure we get enough sleep. A restless night can cause us to feel badly the next day, so a little catch-up time is probably in order. Peaceful sleep any time, day or night, helps us build up our reserves after a bout of illness.

If you are one of those individuals who simply cannot sleep in the daytime, be sure to get additional rest, limit your physical exertion, and deliberately plan activities that you can do while seated or lying down. Maybe there's a book you've been meaning to read, or a sewing or sit-down fix-it project to do. A bad day gives you the opportunity to still get something done and save your energy as you do it.

Another helpful coping skill involves mindful meditation and surrounding yourself with quiet and serenity. If you're having a rotten day, try to get away from noise and bustling activity. Grandkids visiting on one of those days? Run away from home for a few hours if possible. Have some alone time in a quiet room with peaceful music, watch a movie on video or DVD, or just drive to the beach or other serene, scenic place, if you can.

Mindful meditation is not hard to do, it simply means emptying your mind of all extraneous thoughts and focusing on your body to help you quiet the pain. Deep breathing will get you to the right point of concentration. If you haven't mastered this magnificent tool of relaxation yet, give it a try.

Watch your diet on the bad days. Avoid gassy foods such as carbonated soda, beans, and Brusselssprouts. The gas pushes up on your diaphragm, making it even harder to breathe. If you're not on a fluid restriction because of your heart, drink plenty of fluids – water is best – and go easy on the caffeine. If you tend to retain water in your feet and ankles, ask your doctor if you should sit with your feet propped up for fifteen minutes or so, a few times on that day.

Eat regular, balanced meals, even if they are small ones. And be sure to take your medications as prescribed. If your doctor's order is to use your nebulizer or fast-acting rescue inhaler up to four times a day, but you don't usually need it, this is a good day for it. Open up your lungs as best you can. They're telling you they need it!

Save multiple projects for the good days that will surely follow the bad ones. It isn't wise to tax your already stressed system by trying to keep too many balls in the air at once. It's hard enough to juggle time and needs, even when you feel pretty good.

Lastly, deal with your bad days by seeking ways of bringing joy into your life. Find things that make you laugh. Dr. Bernie Siegel, surgeon and author, advises us to handle chronic illness more effectively by creating every opportunity for laughter we can. It's hard to feel bad when you have tears of laughter rolling down your face! If you find joy in listening to music, take time for it. Music can be a wonderful diversion from having to labor for each breath.

Those good days are not far away. If we can just get past the bad ones that loom over us now, things will surely improve. So grab that favorite pillow, the teddy bear you don't let anyone know about, a good book, or a funny movie, and tuck in for a healing time. Do it before you get those eyes-to-the-ceiling looks from those around you – before you affect *their* day. Calmly state that you're having a bad day and hope they will accept that. And work to make your life more bearable right then and there!

Here's wishing you far more good days than bad ones!

Bonus Box I
How the Weather Affects Breathing
JMM

When the COPD patients in Respiratory Therapist Sandy Wright's pulmonary rehab class were discouraged about having "bad air" days, Sandy put them to work…not with a new routine on treadmills and bicycles, but in a much different way.

She began by explaining that the weather can have a lot to do with bad breathing days, and to help them see this for themselves, she engaged them in a study. "I told them to watch the local news every day and track the humidity, the barometric pressure, and the dew point, and also to document how they were breathing on that day."

"Some of my patients were more affected by the humidity while others were more affected by the dew point, which they were surprised The higher the dew point, the harder it was to breathe even if the other [weather] indicators were within normal limits."

"So that was it in a nutshell. After this, they better understood that weather had something to do with their breathing, and they could plan their day accordingly and not get upset if they were having a bad breathing day. They knew it would pass and it wasn't that their disease state was getting worse."

Bonus Box II
Morning Body Scan – Mindful Meditation
JVT

We just talked about ups and downs – good days and bad days – with COPD.

To make those bad air days as good as possible we must to learn to go with the flow, listening to our bodies. Positive attitude helps to even out the peaks and valleys of energy and wellness, but communicating with our inner self is the best way of tuning in to see what's in store.

There is an art to listening to the status of our bodies – Mindful Meditation. We can tap into the state of our bodies before we even rise out of bed in the morning. Here's something that works for me, and I recommend you give it a try. *As always, check with your doctor to make sure that any new physical activity is safe for you.*

When you awaken, take a few minutes to stretch like a lazy cat, reaching your hands high over your head and pointing the tips of your toes downward.

Repeat this action a couple of times with pursed-lip breathing.

Then start to relax and close your eyes again – don't fall back asleep! Breathe deeply and steadily; focus on your breathing. When you feel nice and relaxed, center your attention on the tips of your toes. Visualize first your toes, then slowly your entire feet, as being free of pain and stiffness.

Work your way up with your mind focused next on your ankles, then your calves. In your mind, breathe any pain or stiffness right out of them. Spend a good bit of time thinking about your knees; the joints just may need extra concentration.

Slowly scan your body as you work your way up to the top of your head. Leave no major muscles, bones, and joints untouched by your scan. Just like an X-ray or an MRI, you can examine your body a little bit at a time to check for illness or pain. Then visualize each stopping place as the spot to rid yourself of pain, or at least acknowledge that it is there to be dealt with.

You may find you'll need a lot of practice to become proficient with mindful meditation. That's okay. The better you get at scanning your body in your mind, the quicker you can ascertain your good day / bad day status.

My friends, remember this: If you find, after your morning body scan, that you are headed full tilt for a bad day, it doesn't mean that you must give in to its demands. You don't have to like it, but you can co-exist with a bad day. Instead of being angry and fighting it, simply recognize that it exists. Finally, know that a positive attitude goes a long way toward easing your way through until you wake up tomorrow, hopefully to a better day.

Your Turn

Key points, or ... If you don't remember anything else from this chapter, remember this:

- Frustrating as it may be, good days and bad days without reason are a fact of life with COPD.
- When having a "bad air" day always check for early warning signs of a lung infection (chapter September – Week 3).
- Don't push yourself on the bad days, but take it easy, even if you have to postpone plans.
- Do something enjoyable on a bad air day.
- Tell yourself a good day is right around the corner.

Ask yourself this:

- How did I spend my most recent "bad air" day?
- Should I do something different next time?

This week:

- Set aside fun or interesting projects – something easy you will enjoy doing – for your next bad air day.

Here's more help

- Make a brief call to a friend or log on to an online support group to express that you're having a bad day. Keep it brief. Your friends with COPD will understand and help you get through it.

- http://www.breathingbetterlivingwell.com/community.php
- *Breathe Out: Living Life to the Fullest With COPD, Emphysema or Smokers' Lung,* by Mary Callahan.

Panic and Anxiety in COPD

[Vijai Sharma, Ph.D.]

The first rule is to keep an untroubled spirit. The second is to look things in the face and know them for what they are.
– Marcus Aurelius

Anxiety and panic is common in COPD. In fact, there are some estimates that symptoms of anxiety and / or panic may be experienced by up to 47% of people with COPD[4]. Let's start with looking at some comments from people with COPD who have had problems with anxiety and/or panic attacks. Perhaps you'll find something that sounds familiar. (In order to protect their identity, assumed names are used.)

> I must be having some sort of breakdown as I am constantly sad, worried, and live in fear each and every day. I fear getting up each morning because I am fearful of feeling not well again. I cannot enjoy my family as I feel I am not part of their life anymore, because I am always not well. I cannot enjoy food or social life. I have become almost reclusive as I fear becoming breathless and spoiling my partner's enjoyment. I find myself constantly holding my breath and fear that my COPD is raging on. The more breathless and anxious I feel, the more I

4. Anxiety and depression in patients with chronic obstructive pulmonary disease (COPD). A review. Mikkelsen RL, Middelboe T, Pisinger C, Stage K, Nord J. Psychiatry 2004;58:65 Oslo. ISSN 0803-9488.

notice myself holding my breath. I feel there is no quality of life.

Sorry for moaning but I can't seem to get in control. Exercise is proving difficult as I am anxious of becoming more breathless, which in turn makes it harder for me to manage my life. I fear living, as I feel very isolated and trapped in this body that doesn't work. My aim is to try to be more positive and take each day as it comes, and focusing on my self and my well-being, hopefully without fear.

Julia

I think my panic attacks result from not getting enough oxygen in my system. Don't confuse this with a normal person panting for breath and hyperventilating. Not the same thing. Panic and anxiety is the feeling I have when I can't get my breath. Then I begin to tense up, feeling overwhelmed, jittery and very nervous.

John

My heart races, I get sweaty and I am short of breath when I move around. I am on O_2 when I am up doing things. I sometimes wonder if it is possibly atrial fibrillation [irregular heartbeat]? Should I get a sleep study done or ask my doctor if I should wear a holter monitor for twenty-four hours or more? My friend told me I may even need an "event monitor" to monitor any suspicious heart activity. Could it be a combination of all the meds I take? I do try to stay calm and use the PLB (Pursed-Lips Breathing). Sometimes it works and sometimes it doesn't. What else I can do?

Don

My O$_2$ sats (oxygen saturations) go up and down. I
am now on O$_2$ at bedtime and lately when I am out
and about I am getting these really bad panic attacks.
I wake up in the middle of the night with panicky
feelings and have a hard time trying to fall asleep. Is
there anything I can do to lessen these feelings?
Rodney

COPD has many faces. Yet, there are challenges,
doubts, hopes and fears we all share. John may have a
tendency to be more anxious than Don. Julia might have
had an anxiety disorder before she was ever diagnosed
with a breathing disorder. Don might have more concerns about his COPD symptoms or other symptoms
related to other medical conditions, than Rodney.

Two people with the same degree of shortness of
breath (SOB) may differ with regard to the extent it both-
ers them. One person might say, "I am having trouble
breathing" while another may experience an alarming
sensation, "I will die of suffocation." Each will store these
experiences in their memory differently, setting different
levels of apprehension and anticipatory anxiety.

One might remember it simply as a discomforting
experience, which is a nuisance that can be managed.
Another may remember it as "I could have died," or "I
felt I was going to die. I never want to go through that
again." Some, when anxious, hold their breath or start
breathing rapidly; and some seem to feel the chest tightening and throat closing more than others do. These are
all variations of normal human response to our perception of danger or threat of harm.

Having anxiety, as well as depression, does not mean
you are "weak" or "going crazy." Actually, the presence of
anxiety or depression shows, simply, that you are human

and react like a normal human being. Seeking help or accepting treatment does not mean, "I've lost control, I have failed," or "I am falling apart." Seeking help when one needs it is the wise thing to do.

COPD, with or without anxiety or depression, can also affect family relationships and participation in social life; even leading to isolation from partner and family and losing all interest in relating to others.

There is help and hope! Below are some things you can do if you experience panic and anxiety with COPD.

1. Make sure you have been tested thoroughly for lung function and heart function.
2. When you and your doctor know the physical cause of your discomfort and have taken the necessary steps to regain and maintain your health, you may need an assessment for anxiety, and then learn coping skills. Discuss this with your doctor and be honest about how you feel.
3. You may benefit from anxiety reduction breathing techniques, such as Pursed-Lips Breathing (PLB) and abdominal, or diaphragmatic (DB), breathing. These techniques should be taught by a respiratory therapist or a physical or occupational therapist specializing in respiratory issues. Learn these techniques and use them to manage and control anxiety.
4. Physical and mental relaxation can be a powerful tool for dealing with breathlessness and anxiety. Learn relaxation skills. Relax tense muscles, panicky thoughts, and an anxious mind.
5. Ask your doctor if you might talk to a counselor or other mental health specialist. It is not a sign of weakness to talk with someone about issues

that affect your health, happiness, and well-being. Ask, also, if taking an anti-anxiety medication might help.

Panic and anxiety are common in people with COPD. Breathlessness can cause anxiety and anxiety can increase breathlessness. The more anxious we feel about breathing, the worse the breathlessness gets. But help is available, and there is a lot you can do to feel better if you feel panic and anxiety with COPD.

Excerpted with permission from *Overcoming Anxiety and Depression and Breathing Correctly in COPD/Emphysema: A Self Care Book for People with COPD and a Psychosocial Manual for Professionals* by Vijai Sharma, PhD, intended for future publication.

Your Turn

Key points, or … If you don't remember anything else from this chapter, remember this:

- It is normal to have feelings of panic and anxiety with COPD.
- Reactions to feelings of panic and anxiety differ from person to person.
- Make sure you and your doctor have ruled out other physical causes, such as heart disease, which can also cause panic and anxiety.
- Learning correct breathing techniques along with other treatments and methods can help control panic and anxiety in COPD.

Ask yourself this:

- Do I sometimes feel panic and / or anxiety because of my COPD?
- If so, what happened the last time I felt this way?

This week:

Plan and practice what you will do if you have an episode of panic and / or anxiety. If you don't know where to start, ask your doctor for ideas and references.

Here's more help

- Mind Publications http://www.mindpub.com
- *Working With Asthma, COPD and Respiratory Challenges,* (Mindful Healing) Audio CD.
- *The Miracle of Mindfulness,* by Thich Nhat Hanh.

Panic Attack!
The Anatomy and Physiology of a Panic Attack

[Vijai Sharma, Ph.D.]

*It's not so much what we know as how well
we use that which we know.*
– Ernesta Procope

*This is not intended as medical advice. Show this
information to your doctor. Together you can develop
a plan that works best when you begin to feel panic
and anxiety with COPD.*

What causes a panic attack? What actually happens – physically – prior to and during a breathing panic attack? In this chapter we're going to talk about the physical experience, how symptoms are interconnected, and what causes symptoms to escalate into a full blown attack. Once you understand how a panic attack starts and builds, you will hopefully be able to forestall the onset, or at least modify the intensity of symptoms. As you acquire further knowledge and skills in this area, you may be able to stop them altogether.

A panic attack is nothing but the body's emergency system at work! This is the emergency system that swings into action by an alarm (often a false alarm) set off by your brain. Breath dysregulation (problem with the regulation of breathing) may be the major reason for setting off the emergency alarm or, let's say, our "panic button."

Because breathing problems are a major part of panic attacks, sorting out what's actually going on is particularly tricky for heart and lung patients. You hear a lot about the anatomy of the lungs: Airways, air sacs, diaphragm, ribcage etc., in connection with breathing. But did you know that breathing involves both the brain and the lungs? You rarely hear about the central and critical role your brain plays in monitoring and regulating breathing. Breathing is absolutely essential for our survival; hence it must be under the control of the "higher ups" – your brain. Let's call this the "central respiratory control system."

Your brain is constantly monitoring your oxygen (O_2) and carbon dioxide (CO_2) levels, and the ratio between the two. If the O_2-CO_2 levels and their ratio go outside an acceptable range, the brain gives distress signals, or sets off the emergency alarm. When this happens, our thinking brain may also get involved – in modifying, or magnifying the problem depending on perception, interpretation, and other thoughts related to the breathing episode.

Recurrent panic attacks may be defined as a "dysfunction of the central respiratory control system." This happens when the areas of the brain involved in monitoring and protecting the airways from acute respiratory danger (such as suffocation) become over sensitized and can react inappropriately. This dysfunction may be temporary or permanent.

Let's explore the mechanisms of how the central respiratory control system may begin to overreact and trigger an emergency response, even though there may not be a real emergency. Below are three popular theories regarding panic attacks and central respiratory control dysfunction.

Brain Suffocation Alarm Theory

The brain is constantly reading oxygen and carbon dioxide levels to protect you from suffocation. When it determines O_2-CO_2 are at unacceptable levels, the brain sounds the emergency alarm. Emergency operation, the body's fight-flight operation, swings into action releasing adrenaline, accelerating heart and lung activity, creating hot flashes, cold chills, and hundreds of other changes that prepare us to either fight the problem or flee from it. This emergency action, the "fight-flight' reflex, is what we experience in a panic attack.

The brain constantly checks our blood to be sure also that we are breathing nontoxic air. If it senses a problem, our brain alarm wants us to run away from the dangerous situation. With COPD, even small changes in the air such as odors, pollutions, pollens, sudden temperature changes, emotional excitement, and hurrying can trigger false suffocation alarms.

Hyperventilation and Hyperinflation Theory

Some people tend to mildly hyperventilate (breathing too fast) often. I call this "over-breathing." Over-breathing can create unacceptable levels of the O_2-CO_2 ratio. When this happens, the body's emergency system takes over, resulting in a panic attack. Over-breathing causes the lungs to hyper-inflate, which means that the lungs are not able to get rid of the excess air they are taking in.

Since the stale air doesn't get out of the lungs, there is very little room for the fresh air to get in. When this happens, you try even harder to take in more air and as a result, you feel out of breath. You are unable to "catch your breath." You become hungry for air. Panic sets in.

Catastrophic Theory

Here we rise beyond the territory of the brain and enter the corridors of the mind. Note that our thoughts, also, can trigger the fight-flight reflex. Theory says that when you think such catastrophic thoughts as, "I may never be able to catch my breath and I'll die," or "I might be having a heart attack and I might not make it to the hospital," they can signal the brain of an impending danger and set off the body's emergency alarm system.

These theories offer some insight into how body, breath, and mind interact in a crisis to trigger a panic attack. However, quite often, the perceived crisis is not always a real crisis, but an exaggerated view of uncomfortable body sensations further confounded by our catastrophic thoughts.

In light of the above theories, we can now list the various panic attack symptoms in three categories:

1. Breath-related discomfort
2. Uncomfortable bodily sensations
3. Catastrophic thoughts

We will now classify the thirteen (13) panic attack symptoms in the above three categories:

1.) Breath-related discomfort
- Shortness of breath, smothering
- Feeling of choking
- Dizziness or lightheadedness, fainting feeling

2.) Uncomfortable bodily sensations
- Palpitations, pounding heart, accelerated heart rate

- Chest pain, chest discomfort
- Sweating (not due to heat or exertion)
- Trembling or shaking (in the extremities or the insides)
- Numbness or tingling sensations (parts of the body or the whole body)
- Chills, hot flashes (parts of the body or the whole body)
- Nausea, abdominal distress
- Feeling of unreality or of being detached from self

3.) Catastrophic thoughts
- Fear of losing control or going crazy (e.g. "I'm losing my mind!")
- Fear of dying (e.g. "I won't make it to the hospital!")

Many cognitive therapists believe panic attacks occur due to our highly exaggerated response to breathing discomfort and unpleasant bodily sensations, along with catastrophic thoughts that cross our mind at that time.

I hope this helps you understand how panic attacks can start and build. Talk with your doctor about this so next time you will be able to recognize a false alarm and work your way through it, or understand dangerous symptoms and get the treatment you need.

Your Turn

Key points, or . . . If you don't remember anything else from this chapter, remember this:

- Knowing what is going on physically helps in dealing with feelings of panic and anxiety in COPD.

- Your brain constantly monitors your oxygen (O_2) and carbon dioxide (CO_2) levels.
- The brain sets off alarms that are sometimes only false alarms.
- Understanding symptoms of panic attacks can help you to keep them from taking over and causing a full-blown panic attack.
- It is important to show this chapter and your written answers (below) to your doctor and discuss what symptoms – in your case – may indicate the need for immediate medical attention.

Ask yourself this – write down your answers:

Which of the three theories (Brain Suffocation Alarm, Hyperventilation and Hyperinflation, Catastrophic Thoughts) most applies to me?

_____

_____

_____

Out of the three "Breath-Related Discomforts," which one(s) do I experience?

_____

_____

_____

Out of the eight "Uncomfortable Bodily Sensations," which one(s) do I feel?

_____

_____

_____

Of the two "Catastrophic Thoughts," which one(s) do I have?

_____

_____

_____

This week:

- Remind yourself that not all alarms signal an actual emergency.
- Make a note to discuss this with your doctor at your next visit.

Here's more help

- Mind Publications http://www.mindpub.com
- http://www.breathingbetterlivingwell.com/ articles
- *Psychological Management of Physical Disabilities,* by Paul Kennedy.

Excerpted from the book "Overcoming Anxiety and Depression – Breathing Correctly in COPD/Emphysema: A Self Care Book for People with COPD and a Psychosocial Manual for Professionals, "intended for future publication. Copyright©2008, Vijai Sharma,PhD. (all inquiries to be directed to dr.sharma@mindpub.com)

Accentuate the Positive –
Every Day is a Gift
[JVT]

If you expect nothing, you're apt to be surprised.
You'll get it.
– Malcolm Forbes

Even if we're doing all the right things – taking our medications, exercising regularly, eating right, and getting enough sleep, there is an all-important element for being pro-active in disease management – and that's maintaining a positive attitude. I'm not saying that our disease is only in our minds. We all know this is not the case. However, I do believe that the mind has a powerful influence over the body, and that a negative focus will surely shorten our lives!

We all know too, that COPD can take a terrible toll on us. Each day presents a new set of demands or adjustments. Most of us do learn, eventually, how to live with those physical limitations. But, even if we've modified our activities because of physical limitations, we seem to have an even more difficult time adjusting our mental and emotional outlook.

Maintaining a positive self-image and trying always to look on the bright side can help us heal faster, cope with problems more effectively, and make adjustments for a good quality of life. So, how do we do this? My own approach is simple. *I face each day as a precious gift.*

The gift of a new day is the best one we can receive – a brand new twenty-four hours – 1,440 minutes we've never

ever had before. Think about it. It's like getting God's okay to have another go at it. Each new sunrise dawns like a blank canvas. We can paint the day grey, or we may choose the light, bright hues, and unwrap the hours of each day with the anticipation of wonders and joy to be found.

Focus on the things that you can still do, not on the things you can't. Take pleasure in the small things, find peace and serenity in the goodness that is around us; a child's smile, a mockingbird's song, a neighbor's good deed, time spent with a photo album or journal – all treasures to be found throughout our day.

The essence of good emotional health is to maintain a positive attitude in this way while still knowing the facts and being realistic. Below are some steps we can take to protect ourselves from becoming stuck in the stresses and strains of our limitations. They may seem obvious, but sometimes the simplest things are easy to forget, or taken for granted, so call this a short refresher.

Use the following as a checklist for your own positive attitude. Look it over – every day if you have to – so you can have more control over your life and greater confidence as you face each fresh day.

* Keep learning about lung disease. Read articles, attend pulmonary events, go to reputable websites, and visit the library. The more you know about your disease, the better you will be able to manage it!
* Follow your doctor's orders. Develop a good rapport with your pulmonary specialist. Ask questions when you don't understand something – or if you disagree with the treatment plan. Know your medicines and what they are for. Take them as directed.

* Become part of a breathing support group. You can find them locally and / or online. There is so much we can learn from one another. Go to meetings. Take in the information. Share your own experiences. Make new friends. And most importantly, give each other support! Only others with COPD can know exactly what you are feeling. Healthy people, including our family members, can only assume.
* Maintain an exercise routine. Even a slow and easy exercise program that is followed consistently can help you stay as fit as possible. Do what you can, and with your doctor's advice, keep striving to increase it little by little.
* Smile. At least five times. Every single day.
* Be as active as possible. Fill your life with joy by engaging in activities you love. Find hobbies. Surround yourself with people who care about you, and with whom you can always find something to discuss. Getting out and about requires effort, but we should try to meet that challenge and seek out events and activities that are enjoyable and fulfilling.
* Don't be too hard on yourself. You're only human. If smoking caused your COPD, for example, let go of the guilt and shame. What's past is past. You can't change it now and dwelling on it will only drag you down.
* Keep your sense of humor! Find a joke or funny cartoon each day, and then share it with somebody. Laugh whenever you can – loudly, softly, chuckle, guffaw, or a plain ole' horse laugh. Give it your best shot.

* Focus on what you still can do, rather than what you can't do.
* Only you. Remember that no one else can do these things for you! You, and only you, can breathe for yourself. And you and only you can choose your attitude.
* Look at each day as a gift. Accentuate the positive and never underestimate how that can make a much brighter day for you! Today is a gift. Your gift. Untie the ribbons.

Your Turn

Key points, or... If you don't remember anything else from this chapter, remember this:

- Having a positive attitude can make a difference in not only your emotional, but physical health.
- You can choose your attitude, even if you have severe COPD.

Ask yourself this:

- Have I smiled or laughed today?

This week:

Write down at least one positive event from each day – such as your favorite sports team won a game, a flower bloomed in your yard, or you heard a bird chirping. On the seventh day look back on your list and realize that all those good things happened in your life this week.

Sunday _____

_____

_____

Monday _____
_____
_____

Tuesday _____
_____
_____

Wednesday _____
_____
_____

Thursday _____
_____
_____

Friday _____
_____
_____

Saturday _____
_____
_____

Here's more help

- Maintaining a Positive Attitude While Chronically Ill (author maintains anonymity): http://www.snoskred.org/2007/12/maintaining-a-positive-attitude-while-chronically-ill.html
- *Attitudes of Gratitude: How to Give and Receive Joy Every Day of Your Life,* by M.J. Ryan.

Travel with COPD and Oxygen
[JMM]

The man who has done nothing but wait for his ship to come in has already missed the boat.
– Anonymous

If you have COPD travel might seem to be a thing of the past. But it doesn't have to be that way. While a last minute trip may not be possible, a well-planned one is doable. Whether you choose to take a car trip with a destination close to home, a flight, or a cruise on the other side of the world, you can make it happen – if you know how to prepare and give yourself plenty of time to plan ahead.

If you follow these suggestions, you'll be well on your way to having a healthy and easy-breathing getaway. This is by no means a complete list of travel tips for COPD, but it's a start.

Talk With Your Doctor

The first thing to do is to be sure you're healthy enough to travel away from home. Check with your physician.

Make specific notes outlining the plan you've already made with your doctor about what to do in case of emergency (See chapter September – Week 3 – Preventing Exacerbations and When to Call the Doctor).

If you're going away for an extended period of time, say, a month or more, you may need a referral to a pulmonary doctor at your destination. Folks who participate in pulmonary rehab near their seasonal homes are often required by those programs to have a local doctor.

Know the location of the hospital emergency facility nearest your destination. Not that you'll need it; this is just a precaution.

If you'll be visiting a region with a significantly different altitude and / or climate than you're used to, ask your doctor how it might affect your breathing, then take the steps necessary to make sure you'll still be able to breathe well.

Medications

Obtain whatever prescriptions you need for the entire time you'll be gone, with a couple days extra, in case of a travel delay (or in case you're too tired to go to the pharmacy when you get home). This should include one for an antibiotic and another for oral prednisone, in case of an exacerbation.

If you must fill prescriptions while you travel, working with a nationwide pharmacy (such as Walgreen's or Rite Aid) will make this easy.

Carry with you copies of your prescriptions, as well as a complete list of all the medicines you're on: Name of medicine, dose, and how often you're supposed to take it.

Even if you don't routinely use a rescue inhaler, make sure you have one handy (with spacer or holding chamber). Check to see that it works properly and has enough puffs for eight per day, for as many days as you'll be away.

Keep your medications and paperwork with you, within reach, at all times – in a purse, backpack or tote. Never put them in your airline checked baggage!

Health Insurance

If you have health insurance other than Medicare, check for coverage at your destination.

As you go:

Keep hand sanitizer close by.

Drink plenty of water if your doctor has not given you a fluid restriction.

Stretch your arms and legs at least every hour or two. This will help avoid painful cramps – and life-threatening blood clots! If you're traveling by car, get out and walk around. If you're traveling by plane, train, or bus, get out of your seat and walk up and down the aisle; or at the very least, march in place, lift your legs, or pump your feet on the floor – alternating toe, heel, toe, heel, toe, heel.

Make sure you have access to handicap (or very close) parking at your destination.

Arrange for a hotel room that is accessible without stairs.

Always specify non-smoking accommodations.

Don't plan two big sight-seeing days in a row. The restful day you have in between will be well worth it, even if you have to miss something.

Oxygen

Life is a bit more complicated if you require supplemental oxygen (and we say supplemental because we *all* need oxygen), but don't be daunted by the logistics of arranging a trip. It is possible!

Start by calling your local oxygen provider, tell them where you're going and ask them what arrangements they can make for you. Check with your pulmonary rehab staff and classmates and ask what they know works and what doesn't. Your peers who have traveled with oxygen are a wealth of information; you can learn from their mistakes and their successes.

Unless you're traveling by car, you must call ahead of time (one month is best) to the airline, cruise company, train or bus company, to advise them you'll be using your oxygen. Ask if they require paperwork, such as a doctor's prescription.

Traveling by:

Air – Ask your oxygen provider about renting a portable oxygen concentrator. If they don't have information about it, ask your respiratory therapy professional at pulmonary rehab, your local Better Breathers' Club, or online breathing support group. If you'll be taking a personal oxygen concentrator aboard an airplane, you will need to complete specific paperwork ahead of time. Ask your oxygen company, as well as the airline, what forms you'll need. Your doctor is busy, so allow enough time to have him or her complete and sign the paperwork.

Car – Buckle your oxygen container securely in the seatbelt, making sure your tank oxygen doesn't roll around, and that your liquid oxygen stays upright and doesn't tip over on its side.

Cruise Ship – With the same precautions as above, you can enjoy a cruise even if you're a user of supplemental oxygen. One option is to book a cruise especially for pulmonary patients (See "Here's more help" at the end of this chapter).

Don't Give Up on Getting Away!

So many little details. Is it worth the trouble? Many folks with COPD will tell you that the trip – and the memories – are well worth it!

Allow yourself time to plan ahead, follow these suggestions, learn from others who travel with COPD, and ahhhhh... relax and enjoy your vacation! Don't let COPD cut you off from things that bring you joy. A trip might be just the thing to brighten your life. Happy travels!

Your Turn

Key points, or…If you don't remember anything else from this chapter, remember this:

- It takes some extra planning, but traveling with COPD and supplemental oxygen is possible!
- Check with your oxygen provider about making arrangements for you.
- Talk with your respiratory therapy health professionals (in Pulmonary Rehabilitation, Better Breathers' Club or the staff at your local hospital) about your plans.
- Talk with reliable peers who have traveled successfully – and benefit from their experience.

Ask yourself this:

- If I'm not traveling as much as I'd like, is it my COPD that's holding me back?

This week:

- If you're thinking about taking a trip, ask your doctor if you're well enough to go and if so, take another look at the checklist.

Here's more help

- Sea Puffers Cruises – for people with chronic lung disease and / or supplemental oxygen. http://www.seapuffers.com 866-673-3019.
- Information about getting around with oxygen http://www.portableoxygen.org

A Look at the Lungs
How are They Supposed to Work and What Went Wrong?
[JMM]

If it is to be, it is up to me.
– Anonymous

This week we're going to take a look at your lungs and how they work. Your lungs are complex, intricately constructed, and delicate – yet powerful and tireless in the performance of their duty. Your amazing lungs are the only internal organs that have direct contact with the environment outside your body. So as they work they must take whatever is in the air we breathe and make oxygen available all throughout your body, while at the same time removing carbon dioxide. And no matter what insults they encounter, they are enormously forgiving, continuing to maintain our very breath...and life.

This is a lengthy chapter. But as a COPD educator I know that a big part of learning to live well with COPD is understanding your lungs, how they are made and how they work. You know what they say about eating an elephant. It can be done – if you do it one bite at a time. I'm here to tell you, you're smart enough to understand this. We'll just take it bit by bit, one step at a time.

To see a drawing of the lungs, go to page 351.

The Lungs from the Outside

We're going to learn about the lungs by following the air as it travels through your respiratory system. But before we venture inside the lungs, let's start by looking at them from the outside.

From the outside, the lungs look like two large cones. Healthy lungs are nice and pink, soft, spongy, and elastic. Looking at the lungs from the outside, you can't see the airways (bronchial tubes). Kind of like when you look at a building from the street, you don't see all the rooms and hallways, the elevators and passageways, the heating and cooling ducts, and all the internal wires and cables. Yet, you know they're in there, because you know that building works.

The same holds true with your lungs. Inside that spongy pink tissue, there are many, many tubes through which your air flows, and there are also tiny blood vessels that carry the blood that carries the oxygen.

So, here we go. We're going to start where the air first enters your body and follow it into your lungs, and all the way through the process of respiration.

The Lungs from the Inside

Upper Airway

Your Upper Airway includes your nose, mouth, the back of your throat (pharynx), and your voice box (larynx). It might seem overly simple to say that air enters your body through your nose and mouth, but although you take that for granted, you must know that the upper airway has three very important jobs to do before the air reaches your lungs. It must be filtered, humidified, and warmed. If it isn't, the air you breathe will reach your lungs as too dirty, too dry and too cold – irritating to your delicate lungs.

Preparing your air

Your respiratory system has built-in methods to prepare the air for your lungs.

Filtering

Your first line of defense is the tiny hair-like structures (cilia) in your nose. These hairs help filter out large particles. Have you ever blown your nose after doing a dirty, dusty cleaning or painting project? If you did and saw what was in the tissue, you found all kinds of nasties caught by the hairs in your nose. Good thing that stuff didn't make it into your lungs!

Humidifying

The inside of your upper airway is lined with a thin coating of mucous. The air you breathe is humidified as it passes over this mucous.

Warming

Normal body temperature is around 98.6 degrees Fahrenheit. Unless you're living in the tropics, the air you breathe is not that warm. As the air you breathe passes through your upper airway, it is warmed up.

Bronchial Tubes

In a normal adult, about six inches past the larynx, the windpipe (trachea) divides into two air passages (bronchial tubes). One bronchial tube leads to the left lung, the other to the right lung. As your air makes its way through your bronchial tubes, it continues to pass over mucus, picking up moisture and keeping air passages humidified. Just underneath this thin mucous blanket are more cilia, millions of them, in fact, that sweep the mucous upward, trapping dust, bacteria, and other substances (the stuff that made it past hairs in your nose or mucous in your upper airway). These bronchial tubes progressively branch twenty-two additional times to form more than 100,000 smaller tubes. The tiniest lung airways are called bronchioles.

Alveoli

At the end of each bronchiole is a cluster of air sacs (alveoli). Each alveoli is only about 0.3mm in diameter and just one cell thick; about the same thickness as the wall of a soap bubble or 1/50th the thickness of tissue paper! Normal healthy lungs have more than 300 million alveoli. In fact, if all the airways and air sacs of healthy lungs were laid flat on the ground, they would cover more than one hundred square yards, larger than the size of a tennis court! That's a lot of alveoli, and a lot of surface area to do your lungs' most important job: Oxygen exchange.

Oxygen Exchange

What is oxygen exchange? Simply, it is the process of getting the oxygen you breathe into your blood so it can be pumped by your heart all around your body; and then getting the carbon dioxide out of the blood and back into your lungs so you can breathe it out.

How does this work? Each cluster of alveoli is surrounded by, and is in close contact with, a network of microscopic blood vessels called capillaries. It is here that your oxygen moves through the thin wall of the alveoli, and into your blood. After absorbing oxygen, the blood leaves the lungs and is carried to the heart. It is then pumped through your body to provide oxygen to the cells of your tissues and organs. As oxygen is used, carbon dioxide (CO_2), the waste product of this process is produced. The carbon dioxide is carried by the blood and transported back to your lungs where it is removed as you exhale.

What went wrong? Why is it so hard for me to breathe?

Dirty lungs

Let's go back to the beginning. Remember the cilia, the little sweepers in your airways that help keep your lungs clean? Cigarette smoke and other irritants in the environment can destroy or paralyze cilia. This causes them to stop functioning and your lungs are not able to clean themselves as they should. When this happens, your lungs have to figure out another way to get rid of excess mucous and that's why you may have a frequent, productive cough.

If your cough produces sputum on most days when you do not have an acute infection, you probably have *chronic bronchitis.*

Hyperinflation

When lungs become damaged from cigarette smoking or other hazards in your environment, the elastic fibers within them start to deteriorate and the lungs begin to lose their elastic recoil – their ability to *get air out* efficiently. In COPD the "O" stands for Obstructive, meaning that you have trouble getting your air *out* of your lungs.

Your lung tissue should be stretchy and elastic, like a balloon. The air in a balloon is expelled easily because the balloon is resilient (it returns to its previous shape and size, even after it's been filled up). When lungs lose their elastic recoil, they become more like a paper bag. A paper bag is not stretchy. When air is inside a paper bag, it does not come out easily. It tends to stay there, unless it is squeezed out, requiring extra work.

Also, when your lungs' elastic recoil diminishes you can develop *air trapping* or *hyperinflation*. This means your lungs actually get bigger than they should be – and stay that way. This leads to trouble because the extra, stale air compresses the good lung tissue, so it can't do its job as it should. When your lungs are too big for the inside of your chest, it's overcrowded in there and your lungs have trouble properly expanding and contracting.

Stretched out alveoli, air trapping, and hyperinflation is *emphysema*.

COPD is a combination of chronic bronchitis and emphysema.

Weak Airways

Another result of loss of the elastic fibers is that the airways lose their integrity, their strength to stay open. When this happens they tend to pinch shut or collapse, preventing air from escaping.

Inflammation and Bronchoconstriction or bronchospasm

Exposure over time to lung irritants can cause inflammation (swelling) inside the walls of your airways. When the inside diameter of your airways is decreased, there is less room for the air to pass through, making it more difficult to breathe. Your lungs are irritated, so the muscles surrounding your airways tend to become squeezed and tightened, also causing obstruction and allowing less air to flow in and out.

Muscles of breathing

Your main muscle of breathing is your diaphragm. It was meant to do most of the work of breathing, pulling on the bottoms of your lungs so air can flow in easily. When your lungs become over inflated your diaphragm, which is supposed to be dome-shaped, becomes flatter, putting you – and your lung movement – at a mechanical disadvantage.

When this happens, the accessory muscles of breathing are called to action. The accessory muscles are the muscles around your collarbone, neck, and between your ribs. The problem is they don't do such a good job of moving the air. Using these muscles to breathe not only takes a lot of energy but it can cause your shoulders and back to become tense, sore, and fatigued. More work of breathing, plus less efficient lung movement, adds up to a whole lot of effort without a lot of results. No wonder it's so hard to breathe! (For more on proper breathing techniques see chapters July – Week 1 and July – Week 2.)

I know some of this is hard to hear. Your delicate lungs that do their job so well, so miraculously, are permanently damaged. It's normal – and it's all right – to be upset when you first hear this. But once you get over the initial shock of learning what you should know, you can settle down and get the information you need to move on and do your best to breathe better every day.

Bonus Box
Oxygen, Oxygen Transport and Restrictive vs. Obstructive Lung Disease.

How much oxygen is in our air?
The gaseous mixture that makes up the atmosphere on earth contains 78% nitrogen, 21% oxygen and the remaining 1% is made up of argon, carbon dioxide, water vapor, and other trace gases.

Hemoglobin and Oxygen transport

If you've ever watched a freight train go by, you know there are many types of cars; Coal cars, tankers, automobile carriers, boxcars, and more. Coal, for example, can only travel in the coal car. No matter how much coal has been mined and is ready for transport, if that train doesn't have enough coal cars, there will not be enough coal being delivered.

It's the same with oxygen. Oxygen can latch onto, and travel on only one type of blood cell – the red blood cell or hemoglobin. This is one of the many reasons it's important to not be anemic and have a healthy red blood cell count.

Obstructive vs. Restrictive

COPD is an obstructive disease, a combination of emphysema and chronic bronchitis. In this type of disease something is obstructing the flow of air out of the lungs; either secretions in the airways, airways that are fragile and collapse easily, or airways that are narrower because something has caused the muscles surrounding them to constrict.

People with obstructive disease cannot easily exhale all their air, leaving too much air in the lungs at the end of exhalation.

With restrictive disease: pulmonary fibrosis, interstitial lung disease, asbestosis, sarcoidosis, etc., the lungs are scarred and stiff. This can prevent full expansion of the lungs and make it more difficult for oxygen to cross over from the alveoli into the blood.

Your Turn

Key points, or … If you don't remember anything else from this chapter, remember this:

- It's important to know how healthy lungs work and what goes wrong when you have COPD.
- You have the right to know this, and you should know and understand it, even if it's hard to hear.
- When you know what's going on inside your lungs, you can do a better job of taking care of your breathing, and doing what you can to stay as healthy and active as possible.

Ask yourself this:

- Do I have a question about how the lungs work? If so, jot it down and ask your doctor, respiratory therapist, or other lung health professional about it.

This week:

- See chapters July 1 and July 2 for breathing techniques designed to help you compensate for some of this lung damage. See chapter July 5, to learn about the variety of breathing medications and how each one works on specific problems in your lungs.

Here's more help

- COPD Foundation http://www.copdfoundation. org/
- COPD Info line 866-316-2673

You're Still You
Renewal and Rediscovery
with COPD
[JVT/JMM]

*The will of God will not take you
where the grace of God cannot keep you.*
– Anonymous

We might say that as people with COPD we have been given a bad sentence, dealt a difficult hand to play. Yet, we have more reasons than just about anyone to seek emotional growth and acceptance, and to do it with grace. Learning to do this leads first to renewal, then to rediscovery. This involves finding again, aspects of ourselves that were always there, allowing us to feel content – even under the stress of chronic disease – and to feel joy with others or simply with ourselves.

Throughout the coping process that comes with any chronic disease, we confront terror, loss, rage – all kinds of emotional pain. But when we are able to face both loss and fear of the unknown, we're on our way to achieving some level of renewal. In finding this strength and facing the dreads of disease we learn that having this disease is not so overwhelming after all.

Renewal is like finding ourselves again. This is our same self but in new circumstances – yes, with constraints to handle, but with the tools to continue regardless of changes and loss of ability to do things we once loved.

Renewal is not passive. It is a changing attitude towards our relationship with COPD, born of all our past struggles. Each day brings new challenges, and through this, we learn to set and reset our priorities in such a way that the limitations of our disease no longer define us.

With renewal comes rediscovery – knowing that we are the same persons we always were. Simply, I'm the same me – but a me with COPD. Instead of focusing on *what our disease makes us,* it can become more a matter of *who do we choose to be,* given our limitations?" Yes, we have a choice! It is entirely possible to be physically disabled, or we may call it "limited," without being emotionally handicapped.

We must separate ourselves from the fact that we have this disease – this COPD – and be creative about adapting, and focusing on pleasure and the things we still *can* do, rather than on our limitations and things we *cannot* do. We should do our best, even, to use some of our energy to help other people, and remain actively involved with living.

We shouldn't judge ourselves too harshly. We should accept our limitations with wisdom, but never stop pushing the boundaries. We should live our lives with few regrets. And then give ourselves credit for the effort it takes.

For most of us, tomorrow must be taken in stride. The ability to connect with ourselves, others, and our environment, outweighs the physical limitations we have. We must forgive ourselves for what may have happened in the past and focus on the joys of rediscovering what makes us unique. When we do this we'll be able to accept our disease, along with the grace to be able to continue in the face of COPD – Renewal and Rediscovery!

Remember Dorothy in the *Wizard of Oz*? More than anything she wanted to get back home – and we all know what she went through to get there! Yet, it turned out she was right there, all along. It was an interesting, and sometimes difficult, journey to realize it, but, she already had – within herself – everything she needed.

It took me some time to reach renewal and rediscovery, but I did. It may take you a while, too, but that doesn't mean you can't achieve it. You *can* renew yourself in spite of your lung disease, and you *can* rediscover your best you.

Your Turn

Key points, or . . . If you don't remember anything else from this chapter, remember this:

- You're not a different person.
- You're still you, even though you have COPD.

Ask yourself this:

- Do you ever feel like you've lost the "old" you?

This week:

- If so, find someone to talk with about it. A friend, clergy, or counselor, who specializes in people with chronic disease.

Here's more help

- *Strong at the Broken Places: Voices of Illness, a Chorus of Hope* by Richard M. Cohen.

Could You Have Alpha-1?

[JMM]

If you do not ask yourself what it is you know,
you will go on listening to others and change will not
come because you will not hear your own truth.
– Saint Bartholemew

It was Mary Pierce's 40th birthday. As she stood in the kitchen her phone rang. It was not a call from a friend to wish her well. It was her doctor – with news for Mary that would change her life.

"I was right," he said. "You have this thing called Alpha-1 Antitrypsin Deficiency. It's inherited."

For years Mary had been struggling with shortness of breath, repeated lung infections, severe, unexplained weight loss, and a major decrease in tolerance for physical activity. And all along she blamed herself.

"When I started getting symptoms, mainly the weight loss and shortness of breath, I thought, 'You dummy, you've got to stop this. No doctor's going to be able to do anything for you until you quit smoking.'"

She flashed back to the time when a friend came to visit from California. It was this friend's idea to go play tennis. After running for just three balls Mary was in trouble.

I thought, "Hey, what's going on here? I can't breathe!"

But at that point she could not admit to herself she had a breathing problem, let alone admit it to her friend. "I faked it and said, 'It's really too hot. Let's not play.'"

Mary's reason for not playing tennis that day was the first in a long line of excuses she made for why she could not do what healthy people usually find easy.

Over the next ten years Mary tried to quit smoking. She took several stop smoking classes, and although she had cut down to around a half pack per day, she continued to smoke. But her breathing wasn't getting any better. She was still losing weight and hiding her increasing shortness of breath from her family, friends, and co-workers, doing everything she could to pretend that it was okay.

"I'm a good Catholic girl. I took all the guilt on myself. I said to myself, 'Don't expect anyone else to help. I've got to do it my own dumb self. My smoking is doing it.' So that's how I rationalized it."

Mary's dad died of emphysema and her mom of lung cancer and emphysema. Her grandfather had also died of lung cancer and emphysema. Both Mary's parents had smoked cigarettes. When aunts and uncles came over to play cards the house was full of cigarette smoke. She started smoking at about age 13, sneaking cigarettes.

You might think that it was, indeed, *all her fault*. Not so. What Mary didn't know at the time was that she had a genetically inherited disorder causing her lungs to lack protection from cigarette smoke and other environmental irritants. The damage was occurring at an accelerated rate and was far more destructive than it would have been to a person with normal lungs. At age thirty Mary had the lungs of an old woman.

"Then one time I was sitting up all weekend, struggling to breathe in the chair, really struggling. I thought, 'Man, if I have to live like this I don't want to live anymore.' Monday morning came and I called the doctor. At that point I weighed ninety-nine pounds. He took one look at me and said, 'You're too young to have this much lung disease.'"

&

Back to where our story began...

The doctor continued, "You have this thing called Alpha-1 Antitrypsin Deficiency. It's inherited. They're doing some experimental treatment at the NIH (National Institutes of Health). We can try to get you into a clinical trial."

"That gave me some hope," said Mary. "Then he said, 'They're also beginning to do lung transplants.' Transplants! That's the one thing that told me how bad it was. (At this point in time, in 1987, there had only ever been one lung transplant done on an Alpha-1 patient in all of North America.)

"I can remember standing in my kitchen, hanging the phone up, and saying to myself, 'OK, what do we do now? What do we do to make this go away?'"

&

Over the following months, in spite of doing all she could to maintain her breathing and her health, Mary's lung function declined to a meager 14% (30% is severe, 25% considered disabled). She was on oxygen full time and had just ordered a wheel chair when she received a phone call that would again change the course of her life. But this time it was good news.

It was the transplant coordinator at the University of Michigan saying they had lungs for Mary. Lung transplant, for any lung disease, is extremely complex and relatively rare. But after an uneventful transplant surgery followed by an unusually successful post transplant course, Mary is still doing well today.

Over twenty years after that fateful phone call, Alpha-1 Antitrypsin Deficiency is still hugely under diagnosed. Awareness is abysmal, even among many physicians and those in the health care community. Patients with Alpha-1 see, on an average, six doctors over the course of several years before being correctly diagnosed. Patients with Alpha-1 are often told they have severe asthma or that they have severe COPD at a young age, caused by nothing but cigarette smoking. The vast majority of people with Alpha-1 do not receive transplants and must live with advanced COPD at an early age.

In spite of progress with increased awareness, dedicated research, and better treatments, we still have a long, long way to go. Finding Alphas early in the course of their disease empowers them to seek the best treatment and stay as healthy and strong as possible. If you have COPD you should know about this genetic disease and ask yourself, "Could I have Alpha-1?"

Alpha Facts

* Alpha-1 Antitrypsin Deficiency (Alpha-1) is a condition that is passed from parents to their children through their genes.
* This condition may result in serious lung and/or liver disease at various ages in life.
* People with Alpha-1 have received two defective alpha-1 antitrypsin genes, one from their mother and one from their father.
* Alpha-1 occurs when there is a lack of a protein in the blood called alpha-1 antitrypsin or AAT.
* The main function of AAT is to protect the lungs from inflammation caused by infection and inhaled irritants, such as tobacco smoke.

* Alpha-1 Antitrypsin Deficiency (A-1AD) is one of the most common serious genetic conditions in America and is more common than Cystic Fibrosis.
* The World Health Organization has recommended that all individuals with COPD and adults and adolescents with asthma should be tested for Alpha-1.
* Alpha-1 can cause liver disease in children or severe liver and lung disease in adults, most often causing early emphysema.
* 25 million Americans are estimated to be genetic carriers of this disorder.
* Alpha-1 diagnosis is often missed, even by doctors.

(*Source: Alpha-1 Foundation http://www.Alphaone. org*)

Your Turn

Key points, or… If you don't remember anything else from this chapter, remember this:

- Alpha-1 Antitrypsin Deficiency (A-1AD) is one of the most common serious genetic conditions in America and is more common than Cystic Fibrosis.
- Alpha-1 is often misdiagnosed as asthma or common COPD, due to smoking.
- Testing for Alpha-1 is done with a simple blood test.
- Members of a vibrant Alpha-1 community are ready and willing to help Alphas breathe better and live full lives.

Ask yourself this:

Could I have Alpha-1?
- Are you age twenty to fifty and short of breath with little effort?
- Did you quit smoking with no improvement?
- Do you have frequent lung infections?
- Do you have asthma, emphysema, chronic bronchitis, or bronchiectasis?
- Do you have a family history of lung disease?
- Do you have cirrhosis of the liver with no history of alcohol?

(Source: Alpha-1 Foundation http://www.Alphaone.org)

This week:

- If you answer "yes" to any of these questions, talk with your doctor about getting tested.

Here's more help

- www.alpha1.org – Alpha-1 Association 800-521-3025
- www.alpha1.org – Alpha-1 Genetic Counseling Center 800-785-3177
- www.alphaone.org – Alpha-One Foundation 877-228-7321
- *Breathe Better, Live in Wellness: Winning Your Battle Over Shortness of Breath,* by Jane M. Martin. In this book you'll find more about Mary Pierce as well as the story of the Walsh family and the Alpha-1 Foundation.

How to be Able-Hearted When You Can't be Able-Bodied

[JVT/JMM]

The question was this: If you could say something to somebody with COPD who was about to give up, what would you say?

A wise lady with very severe COPD answered, "Do something to help someone."

As COPD patients, we go through many changes as our disease progresses. We need to adjust, because shortness of breath and fatigue lead to more limitations and less tolerance for exercise. Over time, these limitations result in a loss of the ability to do many things we used to do. Chronic obstructive lung disease is a persistent illness, one that won't go away, and it has no cure (at least for now).

Knowing all this could result in a terrible loss of self-esteem and independence, causing us to just give up and withdraw from the rest of the world, feeling sorry for ourselves and expecting people to do everything for us. It could – but it doesn't have to.

So, how do we make it through this? It's important that we learn to make adjustments in our lives, follow our COPD management plan every day, accept ourselves as we are, doing what we're able to do – and knowing our limitations. And we have to do this without holding on to the anger or bitterness we may have felt when we were first diagnosed.

The very process of evolving to a healthy emotional state can be daunting. Being emotionally healthy means that we must not judge ourselves, comparing what we do now to our previous physical capabilities. Our bodies may be less able than they were in the past, but our minds are not!

So, here it is – the good news! Even if we're not able-bodied, we can still be "able-hearted." We can discover in ourselves something beyond physical constraints and learn to help others. It might take some creativity, but it can be done. Working from the inside out, we can find ways to live a full and productive life by helping people; knowing that even if what we do seems insignificant, it can have a positive effect on that person, and it can be very rewarding for us.

If you have COPD, even if it is advanced, you can still be useful. Your work on earth is not done. You can help others and discover the reward of knowing you made a difference.

Below are some ways you can be able-hearted:

* Accept yourself as you are now, even though you might not be able to do what you once did.
* Focus on today, not yesterday or tomorrow.
* Learn to ask for – and accept – help when it is needed. Without shame.
* Maintain social contacts with friends and family.
* Take a creative approach to the use of your limited energy.
* Keep a sense of humor and fun.
* Help others. Below are thirteen things (some that take little or no energy) you can do to help

someone. There are hundreds more things you can do. Remember, some of these might seem like nothing at all, but they make a difference... more than you know.

* Smile at someone.
* Say "thank you" with a smile and eye contact.
* Tell someone, "You look nice today."
* Write a thank you note.
* Call a friend to wish them a good day.
* Read to a child.
* Listen to a child read.
* Pray for a friend in need.
* Pray for world peace.
* If you're able, make cookies for someone who deserves a treat.
* Make baby hats or blankets for your local birthing center.
* Perform a small repair project for a friend or neighbor.
* Express compassion (maybe that person is worse off than you are).

Do your best to take tomorrow in stride, whatever it may bring. Be confident that each day will provide opportunities for positive experiences. Expect good things. Don't let the good stuff slip by because you have become entangled in a web of hopelessness and despair.

Forgive yourself for what you can no longer do. Celebrate the things you can do! Search deep inside for the strength – and the heart – to live graciously and with caring. Live each day with no regrets. Do your best with the here-and-now. Don't spend your time and effort longing for things that might have been. Allow yourself to coexist peacefully with your COPD. The ability to be connected to ourselves, to others, and to the world around us far outweighs our physical limitations.

And remember, you are not just a patient with lung disease. You are a complete person. You are able-hearted!

Your Turn

Key points, or ... If you don't remember anything else from this chapter, remember this:

- Even though your physical abilities may have changed, you are still useful and valued.
- Accept yourself as you are.
- In helping someone else, you help yourself.

Ask yourself this:

- What can I do to help someone today?

This week:

- Do at least one thing on the bulleted list.
- What did you do, and how did it go? Write it down here.

Here's more help

- *After the Diagnosis: From Crisis to Personal Renewal for Patients with Chronic Illness,* by Joanne Lemaistre.
- Meeting Life's Challenges http://meetinglife-schallenges.com

Nutrition
[JMM]

Don't dig your grave with your own knife and fork.
– English Proverb

They say, "You are what you eat." It's easy to see why that makes sense when you're trying to lose weight, gain weight, or if you have issues with your heart or your digestive system. But, does what we eat have any effect on our breathing? And if so, how? In this chapter we'll look at some basic guidelines, as well as some questions about proper nutrition with COPD.

Good nutrition is important for everyone, and it's especially important if you have pulmonary disease. Food is the fuel your body needs in order to perform all activities – including breathing. Good nutrition also helps the body fight infections, the very infections that can settle in your lungs and lead to pneumonia. For the person with COPD, shortness of breath can make eating difficult, just when you need to eat well to maintain your health and strength. This week we'll explore ways to eat right and maximize your food intake, to produce energy and stay healthy and well.

Your body uses food for energy as part of a process called metabolism. In the process of metabolism, food and oxygen are changed into energy and carbon dioxide.

Metabolism: Food + Oxygen =
Energy + Carbon Dioxide

Food provides your body with nutrients (carbohydrates, fat, and protein) that affect how much energy you have and how much carbon dioxide is produced. Energy is needed not only to perform activities of daily living but simply to keep our bodies alive. Carbon dioxide is a waste product that leaves your body when you breathe out.

Body Weight

It's important to maintain a healthy body weight. Ask your health care provider or registered dietitian what your "goal" weight should be and how many calories you should consume per day for optimum health.

If you are overweight, your heart and lungs must work harder, making breathing more difficult. In addition, the extra weight might demand more oxygen. To achieve your ideal body weight, exercise regularly and limit your total daily calories. If you are overweight, dropping just 10% of your weight will make it easier to breathe, and take stress off your knees and back.

Being underweight is a serious problem for many people with COPD. This is addressed below, in question number six.

Below are commonly asked questions about nutrition for COPD. You'll note that some of the foods that are recommended as good to eat might also be found on another list of foods to avoid. Not everyone can tolerate every food, so pay attention to what you eat and how it affects you and adjust your food plan accordingly.

1. What should I eat to breathe better?

Eat a well-balanced diet of protein, carbohydrates, fruits, vegetables, and yes, even fats. Eat lean meats, whole grains rather than white bread and rice, and healthy fats such as olive oil. Eat the rainbow – foods with a variety of colors – bright colors (candy doesn't count!). These are foods such as tomatoes, dark leafy greens, carrots, broccoli, squash, red peppers and citrus. If you have a large grocery or farmer's market near you, consider trying one new fruit or vegetable each week. Eat a variety of foods from all the food groups, such as those found in the Food Pyramid, to get all the nutrients you need.

2. **Are there foods I should avoid? Foods that make it harder for me to breathe?**

   Avoid foods that cause gas or bloating. A full stomach or bloated abdomen can make breathing difficult. Not all of the foods listed below cause everyone to experience gas or bloating. Pay attention to what you eat and if it causes problems for you, avoid it and see if you begin to feel better. Foods that are more likely to cause gas and bloating include:
   - Carbonated beverages
   - Fried, greasy, or heavily spiced foods
   - Beans, broccoli, Brusselssprouts, cabbage, cauliflower, corn, cucumbers, leeks, lentils, onions, peas, peppers, radishes, scallions, shallots, and soybeans.

   Don't waste your energy eating foods that provide little or no nutritional value (such as potato chips, candy bars, colas, and other snack foods).

   Avoid eating more than one or two pieces of candy per day.

3. **Why do I get so tired when I eat?**

   You might be eating too fast. You might be slumped over, or you might be talking while eating.

If you become exhausted while eating here are some tips that may help:

- Take your time.
- Chew slowly.
- Put your fork down after every few bites.
- Sit in a chair with good back support and sit up straight.
- Use pursed-lip breathing.
- Choose foods that are easy to prepare so you still have energy for eating.
- Ask your family to help with meal preparation.
- Check if you are eligible to receive Meals on Wheels.
- Freeze extra portions of what you cook so you have a meal already prepared when you're tired.
- Rest before eating so you can enjoy your meal.
- Try eating your main meal earlier in the day so you have enough energy to last you for the day.
- Wear your oxygen while eating.

Remember the formula:
Food + Oxygen = Energy + Carbon Dioxide

(For tips on saving energy with food preparation see May – Week 2 – Making the Most of the Breath you Have – Energy Conservation and Work Simplification – Bonus Box: In the Kitchen.)

4. Why do I feel so full after a meal and find it even harder to breathe?

Over-inflated lungs, found often in COPD, can press down on the stomach. In turn, a stomach distended with food or gas pushes up and compresses the lungs. No wonder it's hard to breathe! Eating frequent small meals – up to six per day – will take up less room in your stomach, can help you feel more comfortable and put less stress on your system.

5. **Do dairy products cause me to produce more phlegm?**

It depends on the person. Some people find that milk and other dairy products tend to either increase the amount of phlegm or make it thicker. If this is your concern, try reducing dairy products. After doing this if you find that your phlegm production or phlegm thickness is reduced, then you should avoid them.

If you eat dairy products, and it does not seem to make your phlegm worse, then it's all right to go ahead and consume them. Again, pay close attention to what you eat, see how it affects you, and if you find that a certain food causes a problem for you, avoid it.

6. **I'm shrinking! How can I gain weight?**

Did you know that the simple act of breathing takes more energy for people with COPD, requiring up to ten times more calories than those of a person without COPD? If you have COPD it's important for you to consume enough calories to produce energy in order to prevent wasting or weakening of the diaphragm and other muscles. Your body needs fuel and if you've run out of fat, your body will begin to burn muscle. Don't burn your breathing muscles for fuel!

Keep in mind that a poor appetite may be due to depression, which can be treated. Your appetite is likely to improve after depression is treated. Ask your doctor about this.

If you're at or below ideal body weight and have COPD, check with a registered dietician about starting a weight gain plan. He or she may recommend you take a nutritional supplement in addition to healthy, high-calorie meals.

Here are a few ideas for snacks to help you gain or maintain your weight.

· Pudding made with whole milk
· Soft or semi-soft cheeses
· Granola bars
· Custard
· Low-salt tortilla chips topped with melted cheese
· Crackers with peanut butter
· Bagels with cream cheese – not reduced fat
· Cereal with half and half
· Fruit or vegetables with dips
· Yogurt with granola
· Dried fruits
· Premium ice cream
· Cookies and brownies
· Popcorn with margarine and parmesan cheese
· Bread sticks with cheese sauce

7. **What's the best thing to drink when you have COPD?**

As much as some of us love our coffee (or our wine!), we must remember that good old water is the best thing we can drink for our health. You should drink at least six to eight eight-ounce glasses of non-caffeinated beverages each day to keep mucus thin and easier to cough up. If you have to get up at night to urinate, drink more of these earlier in the day to avoid extra trips to the bathroom during the night.

8. **What about salt / sodium and retaining fluid?**

We just talked about the importance of drinking fluids, but some people with COPD who also have heart problems may need to limit their fluids.

If you have a problem with swollen feet and legs, it may be due to extra fluid in your body, forcing the heart and kidneys to work harder. One way to keep from retaining fluid in this way is to decrease your intake of sodium, or salt. It is generally recommended that we consume no more than 1500 mg of sodium per day, and less, if you have fluid retention as mentioned above.

It's possible to eat well with a reduced sodium diet. Here are some tips:

• Use herbs or no-salt spices to flavor your food.
• Don't add salt to foods when cooking.
• Keep the salt shaker off your table.
• Read food labels and avoid foods with more than 300 mg sodium/serving.
• Use a salt substitute approved by a registered dietician. There are many choices available.

Monitoring your weight every day is recommended. If you are taking diuretics (water pills) or steroids, such as prednisone, your weight may fluctuate significantly. If you have an unexplained weight gain or loss (two pounds in one day or five pounds in one week), contact your doctor. If you take diuretics (water pills), you might also need to increase your potassium intake. Check with your doctor. Some foods high in potassium include oranges, bananas, potatoes, asparagus, and tomatoes.

9. What about Vitamins and Supplements?

Most balanced diets contain enough vitamins to meet your basic needs. On the other hand, taking a multi-vitamin is considered safe and may be helpful. Ladies, check with your doctor if you should be taking added calcium for strong bones.

Be aware that some diet supplements can interfere with your prescription medications or actually cause health problems. Always check with your doctor before taking something, even if it is a non-prescription or OTC (over-the-counter) product.

10. What about fiber?

Include high-fiber foods such as vegetables, cooked dried peas and beans, whole-grain foods, bran, cereals, pasta, rice, and fresh fruit, in your diet. Fiber helps move food along the digestive tract and control blood glucose levels. A good goal is to consume twenty to thirty-five grams of fiber each day. Here's an example: one cup of all-bran cereal for breakfast, a sandwich with two slices of whole-grain bread and one medium apple for lunch, and one cup of peas, dried beans, or lentils at dinner.

Good food plus oxygen is the fuel we need for energy – and for living!

Modifying your eating habits will not cure COPD, but it can help you feel better.

Show this chapter to a registered dietitian and ask what you can do to eat for your best health. A RD can provide safe, in-depth nutrition guidance and create for you a personal action plan for your best possible nutrition.

Your Turn

Key points, or…If you don't remember anything else from this chapter, remember this:

- Eating right for COPD can help you feel better and breathe better.
- It is harder on your breathing if you are overweight.
- If you have COPD, it is not safe for you to be under what is considered to be your "ideal" body weight.

Ask yourself this:

- Am I doing all I can to eat right for COPD?

This week:

- Keeping with any restrictions or special nutritional guidelines given to you by your doctor, make at least one beneficial change in your nutrition and / or eating habits.

Here's more help

- Cleveland Clinic http://my.clevelandclinic.org/ disorders/chronic_obstructive_pulmonary_ disease_copd/hic_nutritional_guidelines_for_ people_with_copd.aspx
- For tips on saving energy with food preparation, see chapter May – Week 2, Energy Conservation and Work Simplification – Bonus Box: In the Kitchen.

Coping with Stress
[JVT]

*Don't hurry, don't worry. You're only here for a short
visit so be sure to stop and smell the flowers.*
– Walter Hagen

Life with any chronic illness has its share of stress – those
of us living with COPD are prime examples of that. Lung
disease, especially, results in major compromises to our
lifestyles and activities. We may lose our independence,
suffer from periodic bouts of depression, even tend to
isolate ourselves from friends and family – all the time
fighting for our breath! We may feel anxious, nervous,
or overwhelmed. Yes, indeed, I would say that stress is a
regular visitor to those of us with COPD.

What does it take to get through this stress? What
works for one person may not work for the next. We all
need to find the coping skills that work best to bring us
out from under the dark clouds, back to clear, blue skies.
I hope you have some of your own stress-relieving methods. Below are a few of mine. Maybe they will help:

Meditation

A few minutes of quiet solitude can provide me with a
chance to meditate my way free (at least, temporarily) of
emotional – and sometimes physical – stress and strain.
I focus on my breathing, taking deep breaths in and
slowly exhaling until my mind becomes clear of all the
things that have been pulling at me.

Then I guide my thoughts and visualize a soothing, peaceful scene...sometimes it's by the ocean on a warm, sunny day where I can smell the salt air and hear the waves. Other times it's a serene Irish garden by a pond, and I can imagine smelling the roses and freesia as I hear birds singing in the trees. I have many other favorite places to "go" (with visualization) in times of stress. Fifteen minutes of meditation like this will bring me comfort and assurance that I will be all right.

Tai Chi Chuan

This ancient Oriental form of stretching seems to help me drop the weight of worries, especially those caused by COPD. It is a gentle form of exercise that even lung patients can learn and do, and it helps keep my body toned and limber. I practice it a couple of times a week – more if I need it. I recommend tai chi as a wonderful muscle conditioner, especially if you aren't able to engage in a strenuous exercise routine.

Listening to music

Soft, classical music has a calming effect on most people, but whatever works for you is best. I enjoy taking a few minutes with my feet up, listening to quiet classics. I have a CD that has classical music set to the sounds of the ocean – truly the best of all sounds for my ears! Just a few minutes away from the worries of the day brings me peace and contentment.

Playing games

If I need a really strong distraction from stress, I can play against the computer in a game of Scrabble. I'm not brave enough to play real people online, although it can be done. Doing this totally distracts me from obsessing about problems I can't do anything about. A game takes about twenty minutes and I don't have to look for someone who wants to play.

Active exercise

There's nothing like a good walk outdoors (on breathable days) to get rid of the cobwebs in my brain and relieve the stress of COPD. If you can't walk, try exercises designed to help your breathing muscles or to help condition the whole body. Exercise is one of the best stress busters!

Journaling

I recommend this for everyone! You'd be amazed at how much better you feel, and how much the load will have lightened after you've expressed your feelings by writing in your own private journal. For your eyes only, this journal should be off-limits to anyone else. And, oh yes, feel free to write in your journal on the good days, too. It doesn't have to be reserved for just the negative feelings.

As the song goes, "These are a few of my favorite things..." to help me over the humps of bad days, stress and worries. One more thing – it helps to remind myself that the current bout of stress won't last. It makes it easier to know I can work my way through it, rather than let it take me over and control my entire existence. Whatever it is that is bothering me, it doesn't deserve that kind of importance in my life! Or in yours!

My solutions may not be right for you. The important thing is to be aware of the many coping skills available to help us conquer the stress of life with COPD. Make your own list of favorite things, and keep them handy for those days when you're stressed out from dealing with lung disease.

Your Turn

Key points, or … If you don't remember anything else from this chapter, remember this:

- It is normal to feel stress when you have COPD.
- There are many things you can do to control stress.
- It's a good idea to have more than one way to handle your stress.

Ask yourself this:

- Do I have a method for controlling your stress that works for me? (Cigarette smoking doesn't count!)

This week:

- When you feel stressed, write down what you are feeling and why, then try one of the above stress reducing methods. Write down how it made you feel.

  _____

  _____

  _____

Here's more help

- "Manage Your Stress," by Vijai P. Sharma, PhD
  http://www.mindpub.com/art099.htm
- *Coping With COPD,* by Elaine Fantle Shimberg.

The Emotional Impact of Being Diagnosed and Living with COPD
[JMM]

A man who says he has never been scared is either lying or else he's never been any place or done anything.
– Louis L'Amour

Do you remember the day you were diagnosed with COPD? Many people do. Although you might have seen it coming, when you hear the doctor say, "You have COPD, it is in the moderate/severe/very severe stage, [he or she might call it "end-stage"], and there is no cure," it hits you. It hits you hard.

If you think back to when you were first diagnosed with COPD, you may have felt that your whole life, at that moment and in the following weeks, months, or even years to follow, was in a state of upset. You may have felt – or still feel – that your life as you knew it, the plans you had made, have changed. You may even feel as if your life, and your plans, are gone forever.

An American president once spoke about families getting the news that their loved one was killed in the line of duty. He said that we should never toss about casualty facts without thinking about each and every family. When a wife, parent, or other loved one sees those military officers at their front door, their worst nightmare has just come true. *That* is the war to them. *That moment – and their profound, unfathomable loss – is the whole war.* It matters not how many others have received the very same report. With just a few simple words their whole world comes crashing down upon them.

We might say that being given the diagnosis of COPD is similar. For the person with COPD who has received the diagnosis of a terminal disease, their life – their world – at that moment, is spinning out of control. So, what to do?

When it comes to learning you have a chronic, terminal disease, the real help begins in dealing with and coping with disease and with your changed life – your new life – on an emotional level.

The chart on page 103 chronicles the stages of coping with common feelings and emotions related to being diagnosed with COPD. The "Issue" is how you might feel now, or how you've felt in the past. The "Pathway" is a way to work through that issue. It is called a "pathway" rather than a "solution" or an "answer" because it may take a while – maybe a long while – to get from "Issue" to "I Get It." The "I Get It" is what you might say to yourself after you've made your way through the process of coping with the "Issue."

You are unique and you will work through this in your own time. The important thing is that you work through it. Look at the "Take Back your Life" framework. Where are you?

Your Turn

Key points, or … If you don't remember anything else from this chapter, remember this:

- Being diagnosed with COPD will most likely change your life.
- For most people, coping well with the diagnosis and life with COPD is a process and does not come all at once, but in stages.

Take Back Your Life
A New Framework for Living Well with COPD

.www.breathingbetterlivingwell.com jane@breathingbetterlivingwell.com

Copyright Jane M. Martin, 2010

The Issue	The Pathway	"I Get It!"(and I'm going to be okay)
Denial: I don't have COPD or emphysema. I was just fine until I got that last cold. This is just bronchitis.	**Recognition** Recognize the fact that you have COPD.	I may not like it, but I guess I do have this, and at least now I know what I'm dealing with.
Fear: Nobody seems to see what's happening here, so it must be in my head. I can't let this get to me, because if I do, it just means I'm weak—and giving in. But…still…I think I might be losing it.	**Validation** Realize that it is okay—and normal— to be scared about this diagnosis.	I'm not weak, and I'm not crazy. It makes sense for me – or anybody who has this – to be scared sometimes. I'm normal.
Loneliness: I'm all alone. I must be the only one who has this. If there are others, where are they?	**Voice** Know it is estimated that 24 million people in the US have COPD and 210 million worldwide*. There is strength in numbers and those numbers are beginning to be heard.*Source: World Health Organization, 2009.	I am not alone! There are millions of others out there like me.

The Issue	The Pathway	"I Get It!"(and I'm going to be okay)
Confusion: Inhalers, nebulizers, oxygen… this is just too much to take in. I'm constantly confused and overwhelmed and my breathing is out of control.	**Education** Learn all you can about COPD from solid, credible sources. Ask your doctor to refer you to pulmonary rehab.	Now that I understand what's going on in my lungs, I know what I can do to make my breathing as easy as possible. I can do something about it.
Isolation: Nobody understands what I'm going through. They can't possibly understand what it is like to be so short of breath.	**Support** Join a breathing support group, pulmonary rehab, online support group, or all of these	It really helps to talk to and be around others with the same problem. They understand.
Despair: I'm useless. I can't do anything anymore. I'm all washed up. I'm of no use to anyone.	**Service** Do something to help someone, a person with or without COPD.	There are things I can no longer do, but there are many things I can do! My friends, my family, and my community need me. My life has meaning again!

- It is possible to work through the emotional issues and have a full and happy life with COPD.

Ask yourself this:

- Where am I on the "Take Back Your Life" framework? (You might be in more than one place.)

This week:

- If you are in the "Issue" column in any of the six steps, try starting out on your pathway. If you are in the "Issue" column in any of the six steps, try starting out on your pathway. If you are in any of the "I get it!" boxes, good for you! Go down the chart and see how you're doing on other issues.

Here's more help

- *Breathe Better Live in Wellness: Winning Your Battle Over Shortness of Breath,* by Jane M. Martin, BA, LRT, CRT. Stories of people not just surviving, but thriving, with chronic lung disease.
- *The Chronic Illness Experience,* by Cheri Register.
- Breathing Better, Living Well community forum:
- http://www.breathingbetterlivingwell.com/community/index.php
- American Lung Association – Finding a Better Breathers Club in Your Area:
- http://www.lungusa.org/lung-disease/copd/connect-with-others/better-breathers-clubs/
- To contact the American Lung Association nearest you, call 1-800-LUNGUSA (586-4872).

Make the Most of the Breath You Have : Energy Conservation and Work Simplification

[JMM]

Rivers know this: there is no hurry.
We shall get there someday.
– A.A. Milne

Probably one of the most common complaints in pulmonary rehab is expressed in this way: "I can do a lot here. I'm walking for twenty minutes, I'm working with weights and everything. Why do I still get so short of breath when I'm walking out to my car?"

No matter how well someone does in pulmonary rehab or independent exercise – even though they're making progress increasing their walking distance and endurance and improving their strength and flexibility – if it doesn't make a positive difference in their everyday life outside our doors, we've somehow missed the mark.

Learning energy conservation and work simplification tips and techniques forms a bridge from gym to home. It can help you benefit from the gains you make in physical fitness and make a big difference in the way you live, improving your quality of life on a day-to-day, hour-to-hour basis.

Below are some of the basic concepts of energy conservation and work simplifications for people with COPD. Working with a certified Occupational Therapist can maximize your ability to do what you need – and

want – to do in your everyday life with minimal shortness of breath.

* Pace Yourself
  Pacing is one of the most important things to
  learn. In pulmonary rehab, when participants
  talk about what causes them an increase in shortness of breath, something that often comes up is
  "rushing or hurrying." When you have COPD
  with significant shortness of breath, you simply
  cannot rush or hurry.
* Breathe right
  Using correct breathing techniques can go a
  long way in helping you feel less short of breath.
  When you are performing any kind of activity, always exhale during the most difficult
  part; exhale as you lift, bend, or climb stairs. If
  you become short of breath, stop and rest for a
  moment before resuming your activity.
* Listen to your body
  There will be days when you wake up and know
  almost immediately it's going to be a "bad air"
  day and there's no use in denying it. Take it easy
  that day and don't feel guilty about it! (See chapter
  February – Week 3.) Or you may awake feeling
  great and able to do a special task you have been
  saving for a good day. The important thing is to
  learn to listen to your body, trust your instincts,
  and go with them.

Even if you don't go to pulmonary rehab (and I hope you
do!) you can still benefit from learning simple, common
sense techniques. Some of them are things that once you
know, you wonder why you never thought of them before.

Just because you've always done something a certain way, doesn't mean it's a good idea to keep on doing it that way – especially if you're limited by shortness of breath!

Here are a few tips and techniques to help save energy. Once you get used to taking a fresh look at how you do everyday tasks in order to conserve energy, you'll be on your way to better breathing.

* Avoid unnecessary activities

  Ask yourself, "It is really necessary that I do this? What will happen if I don't? Can it wait?" Avoid unnecessary activities that cause you to expend more energy. For example, wear a terry cloth robe after your bath or shower to save yourself the effort of drying off. Allow the dishes to air dry rather than drying them by hand; or better yet, use the dishwasher. If all else fails, delegate.

  Sit, don't stand, to comb your hair, shave, or apply makeup. According to the Canadian Lung Association, sitting uses 25% less energy than standing. Prop your arm up on something when grooming your face and hair.
* Organize your activities

  Plan your most strenuous activities at the time of day when you have the most energy. Alternate between tasks that are difficult and those that are easy. Plan rest periods, knowing it's okay if you need more rest on one day than on another.
* Organize your closets, shelves and drawers

  Place items you use most frequently between waist and shoulder height. This way you won't need to do a lot of bending or stretching to reach them. Keep all items in the area in which they're often used, to avoid extra walking to find them. For example, store living room cleaning products in a basket in or near the living room. Saving steps saves energy.

* Run a fan

    If you are bothered by the heat, use a small portable fan when cooking or ironing. A portable fan is useful in any room, not only to cool you off but to help overcome shortness of breath brought on by exertion or stress. It is also useful for blowing offensive or irritating odors away from you.

* Maintain good posture

    If you use your body properly, you will save energy. Avoid excessive bending or lifting. Use better body mechanics when trying to move items by pushing, pulling, or sliding the item. Instead of carrying things, get yourself a little wagon or cart to wheel them.

* Carry heavier loads close to the center of your body

    Carrying an oxygen tank or heavy purse over one shoulder can cause pain and fatigue, even shoulder injury. When possible, carry items such as this on a strap that goes across your chest or back, using the core of your body to carry the load.

    Ladies, we all love our roomy handbags, but...stop and ask yourself, "What do I really need to have with me?" Maybe you can get by with a simple money clip, tissue, inhaler, and lipstick, in a cute little bag that hangs across your body and rests on your hip. Keys can be clipped to the outside if they're too bulky to go inside.

* Practice relaxation

    When you relax, you help restore energy to your body. Make sure to schedule relaxation periods throughout your day and when doing so, concentrate on relaxing all your muscles and slowing down your breath.

Wait until an hour or more after eating. Digestion draws blood, with oxygen, away from muscles leaving them less able to cope with extra demands. You may find you feel your best soon after taking your medicine or having breathing treatment.

* Supply and demand

When you have COPD you must look at your supply of energy the same as you think of money in the bank. There's only so much of it and it must be spent wisely. Repeated overspending can cause you to experience a deficit in breath. Learning energy conservation and work simplification tips and techniques can make a huge difference in the way you live, so you spend less time huffing and puffing, and more time enjoying life!

Bonus Box

Climbing Stairs – One of the most common problems I hear from people coming into pulmonary rehab is that they become severely short of breath when climbing stairs. Here's a suggested method, but don't try this for the first time when you're alone. *Show this to your doctor or respiratory health professional and ask him or her to work on this with you.*

- Start by holding firmly onto the stair rail. Relax your shoulders and take a nice breath in through your nose.
- Climb the stairs only as you exhale, as you slowly and gently blow your air *out* through

pursed lips (see chapter July – Week 1). If you breathe *in* as you climb, you will tend to hold your breath and that can make your shortness of breath even worse.

· Climb the stairs only as you exhale, as you slowly and gently blow your air *out* through pursed lipsLet's say you exhale for a count of four. In this case, climb just four steps, then stop and take another breath in through your nose and repeat. It may take a little longer to get up there, but you'll reach the top with breath to spare!

In the Kitchen – Food preparation and clean-up can be a big drain on energy and breath. Here are some tips for breathing easier in the kitchen.

· Don't try to do everything at once. Set smaller goals. Almost all jobs can be divided into segments.

· Plan your meals when you are neither hungry nor tired. Eat healthy. Every bite counts. It's too important to leave to impulse.

· Use convenience foods when you have to, but remember that many packaged foods have high salt and sugar contents. Learn to read labels.

· If you enjoy cooking, make double or triple the amount of your favorites. Freeze them and enjoy tasty, easy meals when you need a day off.

· Microwave ovens and slow-cookers make cooking easier and reduce heat in your kitchen.

> - When cooking, always use your exhaust fan, or make sure there is good ventilation.
> - Store your most used pots and pans on the top of the stove. Instead of putting dishes and flatware away, put them near the table, or reset the table for your next meal.

Your Turn

Key points, or ... If you don't remember anything else from this chapter, remember this:

- You can save energy – and breath – if you learn tips and tricks of energy conservation and work simplification.

Ask yourself this:

- What are three actions or activities that I find the most difficult to do?

_____

_____

_____

This week:

- If possible, apply what you've learned in this chapter to save energy. If you don't know how to do this, ask your doctor for a referral to an Occupational Therapist for help, reminding your doc that this will help you remain more independent, and possibly even help you avoid acute exacerbations.

Here's more help

- To find an Occupational Therapist (OT) in your area, contact your local Center for Independent

Living, hospital, or home health agency. Your local yellow pages, also, can tell you if there is a private practitioner in your area.
· Around the Clock with COPD
  http://www.lungusa.org/lung-disease/copd/
  living-with-copd/Around_the_Clock_wtih_
  COPD.pdf
· For more energy conservation tips specifically for:
  Eating – see April – Week 3 – "Nutrition"
  Parties – see December Week 2 – "Nine Ways
  to Help you Breathe Better and Save Energy this
  Holiday Season."

Gardening and Yard Work

[JMM]

(To our friends in the Southern Hemisphere: This week, read
May – Week 3: Facing Fall – Preventing Exacerbations and
when to Call the Doctor.)

[JMM]

*To be surrounded by beautiful things has
much influence upon the human creature;
to make beautiful things has more.*
– Charlotte Perkins Gilman

When new patients come for their first day of pulmonary rehabilitation I ask them about their goals. "What do you hope to improve or change as a result of coming to pulmonary rehab?" Without a doubt, one of the most common goals patients have is to be able to get outside again and work in the yard.

For those unfamiliar with COPD, this might seem simple, but when you're having trouble breathing in the first place, getting outside in the warm weather, moving around, bending over, and lifting, seem impossible. So, how can you, a person with COPD, still work in your yard or garden with enough energy left over to enjoy it?

Here's a true story:

Leona, a patient in our pulmonary rehab program, came in one day really disappointed – and actually quite peeved. She said, "My daughter, Tammy, told me my gardening days are over. Done! She won't let me do it anymore. She says I get too out of breath. That makes me so mad!"

"Oh my," I said. "I know Tammy's just trying to help. She worries about you." I paused. "Hmmmm...I'm sure you can still to do *something* – you just have to know how; pace yourself, and breathe the right way as you work. We'll figure it out."

So I did some research, found some information and gave it to Leona. "Show this to Tammy when you see her on Sunday and let me know how it goes."

We'll get back to the story of Leona and Tammy in a minute, but first, below are some tips on gardening with COPD. Some of this might take a little planning, and a bit of an investment, but it'll be worth it if it means you can work in your yard and still have the energy – and the breath – to enjoy it!

Plantings

* Reduce the total size of your gardening area and flower beds, focusing on your most favorite plants.
* If you become breathless by getting on the ground and bending over, consider replacing areas of your garden with easier-to-reach raised beds.
* Trade your traditional garden for window boxes.
* Decorate your deck, patio, or terrace with container gardens.
* Use perennials that come up year after year without replanting.
* If you have a large yard, consider replacing some of your garden or grass areas with low-maintenance

ground covers or no-maintenance stones or wood chips.

Tools and equipment

* A 50' long nylon garden hose, with its reel, weighs only 2 1/2 lbs. and can be carried in one hand.
* Use lightweight tools that require less energy. Trade in your traditional hoe and rake for smaller versions with extra-long or extendable handles.
* Use a long-handled gripper for removing gardening debris from the ground.
* Keep tools together in a rolling cart to avoid taking extra steps back to get them. If you are able to carry them keep them in a lightweight bucket or basket.
* If bending over cuts off your wind, try gardening sitting down. You can do this by using a lightweight folding stool or a rolling seat with storage inside.

Weather and the Air

* Check your local weather report or the Weather Channel for air quality and pollen forecasts so you can avoid working outside when allergen, pollen, and pollution levels are high.
* Limit your exposure to intense heat and humidity; garden during the cooler times of the day (early morning and late afternoon).
* Know if you are allergic to things growing in your garden and lawn. If you are and don't want to give up your gardening, use a dust mask when you work.

As You Go

* Cut down weeds while they are still small and leave them where they fall. It makes good mulch.
* If necessary, relocate your garden tools and hose closer to your garden.
* Garden in moderation – especially in the spring when you're raking and preparing beds. Do a little at a time.
* Ask for help – whether it's a tray of annuals or a bag of soil or fertilizer, let someone else do the heavy lifting for you. This includes transporting your purchases into and out of your car.
* Gently stretch and warm your muscles before you begin gardening.
* Slow down, relax, and alternate cardio-intensive activities (i.e. reaching, walking) with tasks requiring less exertion.
* Incorporate frequent breaks into your routine to reduce fatigue.
* When you mow your grass, wear a dust mask. Better yet, ask a family member to cut the grass, hire someone to mow the lawn, or trade in your walking mower for a riding mower.
* For small lawns, if you're able, use a push-mower rather than subject yourself to the fumes of a gas mower.

Raising Monarch Butterflies

This is something popular with folks in our pulmonary rehab program. If you can find milkweed, you will probably find Monarch Butterfly eggs, if you know how to look. Caring for and raising a Monarch is easy, fascinating and fun! See resources in "Your Turn" at the end of this chapter.

For the Birds

If you've always enjoyed feeding the birds but it has become too much for you, you can still keep a birdbath. Position the bath near a hose, preferably one with a high-pressure nozzle. All you have to do is spray it with high pressure to keep it clean and make sure it's filled. Thirsty birds will still stop in and you can enjoy watching them splash.

> So, whatever happened with Leona? I'm happy to report that two weeks later she came in to rehab, beaming. "Tammy stopped by yesterday with a bunch of flowers. We're going to plant them in some pots out on the deck. I'll have my garden after all!"
> Leona's garden might be smaller, it might be different, but it's still something she can work on – and enjoy her yard.

I hope this helps. Remember to pace yourself, think creatively, and ask for help when you need it. Happy Gardening!

Your Turn

Key points, or … If you don't remember anything else from this chapter, remember this:

- You can still have a garden, even if you have COPD.
- Finding just one or two tips and techniques you can use, could make a big difference in helping

you continue with the yard work and gardening you enjoy.

Ask yourself this:

- Is there a tip or technique in this chapter I can use to make my gardening easier?

This week:

- Review the list and commit to making three changes that will make your gardening or yard work easier, and your time outdoors more enjoyable this year.

Here's more help

- Weather and pollen reports –– http://www.weather.com
- Raising Monarch butterflies – http://www.joyfulbutterfly.com/articles/monarchindoors.html
- Accessible Gardening: Tips and Techniques for Seniors and the Disabled, by Joann Woy.
- *Accessible Gardening for People with Physical Disabilities: A Guide to Methods, Tools, and Plants,* by Janeen R. Adil.

Exercise
[JMM]

What saves a man is to take a step. Then another step.
– Antoine de Saint-Exupery

Disclaimer: Always consult your doctor before starting an exercise program. The following are basic suggestions for those who have been approved to exercise under the supervision of a doctor or pulmonary rehabilitation professional. This is not intended as medical advice.

If you have COPD and are short of breath, it's a good possibility that the last thing you want to do is exercise. But, of all the treatments for COPD, exercise might just be the one thing that makes the biggest difference in the way you move, the way you view your disease, even the way you look at life.

Being a respiratory therapist working in pulmonary rehab for many years, of course I would love to see every person with COPD go to pulmonary rehab to learn how to exercise safely in a monitored environment. Unfortunately that's not possible, so here are some exercise basics, for your information. Show this chapter to your doctor and ask if it would be appropriate for you to start an exercise routine.

Types of exercise

Stretching and flexibility exercises help improve your posture, movement and breathing. Stretching the right way can reduce or even eliminate muscle soreness brought on by exercise. Flexibility activities can reduce your chance of falls or other injuries.

Strengthening and resistance exercise helps build muscles, improve strength, and maintain bone health. Lifting hand weights, using resistance bands and working with weight machines are good ways to increase your strength.

Endurance and aerobic exercise helps improve the function of your lungs and heart. Walking, biking, rowing, stepping, and swimming, are just a few endurance exercises. When done correctly, this type of training builds stamina and endurance with shortness of breath you can control.

Breathing Techniques

Always use pursed-lips breathing during exertion of any kind, but especially with exercise. Using correct breathing techniques will help you do more while feeling less short of breath. When you are lifting weights, exhale as you lift. Never hold your breath! Always keep your shoulders relaxed and use the diaphragmatic breathing technique if possible. If you become short of breath, stop and rest for a moment before resuming. See chapters July - Week 1 and July – Week 2.

Getting ready

* Dress comfortably in clothes that move with you. Wear supportive shoes that fasten snugly, and socks that cushion your feet and absorb perspiration.
* If you have a quick-acting Beta-2 agonist (rescue) inhaler, ask your doctor if you may use it fifteen minutes prior to exercise to maximize the openness of your bronchial airways.

* If your doctor has recommended you use supplemental oxygen during exertion, ask your O2 provider to set you up with a portable, lightweight system, and make sure you know how long it will last!
* Start slowly, even if you feel you can do more. If you have not exercised in a while you need to give your body a chance to get used to it again. Don't overdo it on the first day. A muscle that may not hurt today might tell you tomorrow loud and clear that you overdid it! In some programs exercise time is increased by one minute each session (under the direction of an exercise specialist) unless a person is able to do more.
* Begin with a three-minute warm-up. This means go slow and easy for the first three minutes. Don't go full out on cold muscles.
* Do cool-down stretches as directed by an exercise specialist. Stretch just until you feel a gentle pull. Don't bounce!
* Let's say you want to walk outside and you know you're able to walk for ten minutes non-stop. In this case you should walk for five minutes, turn around, and go back to your starting point. Check out your walking route ahead of time (driving your car) to see if there are any places to sit down or lean on, if you need to take a break. Don't get stuck somewhere out there with no breath left to get you home!
* If it's okay with your doctor or physical therapist, add weight or resistance training to your routine. Lifting soup cans or bottled water can help you increase your strength.
* Don't exercise on an empty stomach. Have a light meal or a snack before your work out.

Carbohydrates and protein work well. If it is approved for your diet, peanut butter or cheese on crackers or a peanut butter sandwich is good. Add some fresh fruit and eight ounces of water and you're ready to go!

* If possible, exercise in a group or with a buddy. It will keep you motivated, be more enjoyable, and make sure help is there if you need it. If you must exercise alone inside, keep it interesting! Exercise where you can look out a window, watch TV, or listen to music. If you walk outside alone, walk in the daylight and carry a cell phone.

* If you're in a pulmonary rehab program you'll be monitored by the staff to make sure your blood oxygen, heart rate, and blood pressure are at safe levels. If you're exercising on your own, you can monitor your oxygen saturation and heart rate if you have been trained by a specialist in pulmonary exercise.

Check to see if you qualify to participate in pulmonary rehab. Even if you're significantly short of breath and don't think you're able to exercise, you might be surprised at how much you can do. Pulmonary rehab is a great way to learn safe and appropriate exercise, and learn tips to keep you breathing easier.

Your Turn

Key points, or ... If you don't remember anything else from this chapter, remember this:

· People with COPD, even very severe COPD, can and should exercise.

- Exercise improves strength, flexibility, and endurance – and also helps with circulation and feelings of well-being.
- Do pursed-lips breathing with any exertion, but especially during exercise.
- Consult your physician before starting any exercise routine.

Ask yourself this:

- Am I exercising regularly? If not, why not? What's keeping me from doing this?

This week:

- If you are already involved in routine exercise, ask yourself if it's time to increase your time and / or intensity.
- If you're not, ask your doctor about starting a pulmonary rehab program.

Here's more help

- To find the Pulmonary Rehabilitation program nearest you contact the American Association for Cardiovascular and Pulmonary Rehabilitation http://www.aacvpr.org, phone: 312-321-5146.
- Call your local community senior center (even if you're not a senior) for information on low level exercise classes, television shows, or videos.

What Can I Count on Today?

*Better to lose count while naming your blessings than to
lose your blessings while counting your troubles.*
– Maltbie D. Babcock

[JMM}

With twinkling eyes and a happy smile, Josie was a
favorite patient of mine. She carried herself with confidence and grace – yet a bit of mischief – in spite of
severe COPD, and having suffered loss and betrayal in
the past.

"So, how do you stay so cheerful, in spite of your bad
lungs – and everything else?" I asked.

"It's simple, darling. I ask myself every morning, 'What
can I count on *today*?'" Josie uttered the word, "today,"
in a hushed, almost reverent, tone.

I looked at her, puzzled. She told me a story, and I'm
sharing it with you here.

It was four o'clock on a hot summer afternoon in
1962. Josie, a single mom, punched the clock at the
aircraft factory, jumped in her car, and drove off to
pick up her girls.

Her modest wage covered rent, food, clothing,
and gas, but little more. So, although Josie wasn't
able to take the girls out to movies or buy them toys,
with a spark of creativity and a flare for adventure,
she gave them a good life. And today she had a special surprise that she was sure her daughters, Patty
seven, and Bonnie five, would love.

"Let's go girls! We're off to the lake to go swimming!"

The girls were thrilled! That afternoon the three had a great time, playing in the water and swimming until they headed home after seven p.m.

The next day, same as always, Josie picked up Patty and Bonnie after work. "Girls, I have another surprise for you today. We're going for ice cream!"

The girls were not nearly as thrilled at the thought of this as they were with swimming the day before. But on they went to the ice cream shop. Josie reached into her purse for the last of her meager change, just enough to pay for three scoops of ice cream in three waffle cones. Mom and her daughters climbed into the car, eating their treats and heading for home.

Patty and Bonnie sat low in the back seat, sulking. They looked at each other and began to chant, "We want to swim! We want to swim!"

"Girls…"

"We want to swim!" they said, more loudly each time. And they kept it up.

Josie said, "Give me your cones."

The girls continued to fuss. "We want to swim!" The chant went on.

"Give me your cones!"

Quiet now – and a bit confused – they handed their mother their ice cream cones.

With her left hand on the wheel, and her right hand holding two half-eaten ice cream cones, with one swift stroke Josie tossed the cones out the driver's side window.

"Mom! Our ice cream! Why'd you do that?" The girls began to sob.

"Yesterday we swam and we had a wonderful time. Today we can't go swimming. You had a nice treat in your hands but all you could do is complain that it's not what you had yesterday. Forget yesterday and appreciate what you have today."

[JVT]

People with a chronic, progressive, incurable disease learn that life is worth celebrating. As sicker people, we seem to appreciate life more, probably because we realize that good days are precious and the time we have left may be brief.

Still, even if we have been living with COPD for a long time, we may need to be reminded of the joy of just living; even having a sense of wonder for what each new day will hold. Who can tell if this day will provide us with special memories to be filed away to recall later on? What if this is the day when we get a chance to do a good deed for someone in need? What if this is the start of improved health for me?

Who knows? This might be the day that a cure is found for emphysema; when research finally proves that lung tissue *can* be regenerated. Or, more simply, how about I just enjoy my favorite meal this evening?

There are so many ways we can celebrate life, and each of us should have our own list of favorite things to do. Sure, a great time for me might be less than exciting for someone else. But we all know what special things bring a lift to our heart, a little dance to our step.

One thing we can all do to help us celebrate life is to find ways to help others. There is great joy to be found in doing good things. Maybe we can choose a day to bring lunch to one of our fellow COPDers who has been confined to home. Or maybe we can just bake some cookies for a favorite person, or as a way to say a special thank you.

It could be that someone you know would appreciate help with grocery shopping. Or maybe you can drop off a copy of a good book for someone else to enjoy. The list is endless. And it is easy enough to find activities that don't require a lot of physical exertion.

Try to accept each day with the grace of a life well lived. Make the most of its opportunities. Fill in the blanks and voids of your daily existence with positive thoughts and events.

I look back on the prognosis I was given fifteen years ago – two to five years – and I am grateful that I am still alive; still able to contribute to life around me and still able to function in my daily business of living. And I am still able to meet more outstanding COPD people every month; to reach out to each one of you as I write this.

Quality of life for people living with chronic illnesses may be difficult to recognize sometimes, but it is possible! People with COPD, or any chronic disease, learn that life is worth celebrating, and each new day dawns with a whole new world of reasons to enjoy it.

Your Turn

Key points, or . . . If you don't remember anything else from this chapter, remember this:

- People with chronic disease often learn to appreciate each day moreso than those who are well.
- Finding joy in each day enhances quality of life.

Ask yourself this:

- What can I count on today?

This week:

- Find something each day to appreciate, and write it down.

Sunday_____

_____

Monday _____

_____

Tuesday _____

_____

Wednesday _____

_____

Thursday _____

_____

Friday _____

_____

Saturday_____

_____

Here's more help

- *Chronically Happy: Joyful Living in Spite of Chronic Illness,* by Lori Hartwell.
- But You Don't Look Sick
  http://www.butyoudontlooksick.com/about/

Dying with COPD
[JMM]

The question is not how we will die, but how we will live.
– Joan Borysenko

"What will it be like when I die? Will I just struggle for every breath and gasp until I can't get any more air? That sounds like a horrible way to go! That's what scares me the most."

As a respiratory therapist I've heard concerned, frightened – and rightfully so – COPD patients ask these questions many times. I don't have all the answers, not by a long shot, but I am here to tell you this: The answer is "No." If you are an informed patient, dying – whether you have COPD or not – does not have to be about pain and suffering; rather, it should be all about care and comfort, along with dignity and personal choice.

Let's talk about a subject none of us, whether we have COPD or not, no matter how old or young we are, really wants to talk about – our final days of life.

Never say die?

It's important to tell you that my patients in pulmonary rehab are generally the kind of folks who pretty much never say die. They are spunky and spirited even when things get tough. However, many of them do get to the point at some time or another and say, "You know what? I'm just tired. I gave it my all. I far outlived what the doctors said I would. And I am totally at peace with leaving this life."

What about you? If you have end-stage (I hate that term), or very severe COPD with significant shortness of breath, you might be asking, "Is this it? Am I at the end of the road?" Many times patients have come into our program on the first day, thinking for sure that this is "it" – and once they got into rehab they found there are many things they can do to breathe better and live longer.

Is this the "end of the road?"

As you ask the "Is this it?" question, you must ask yourself these questions too:

* Do you have a good doctor who takes time with you and listens to what you have to say?
* Have you and your doctor discussed, and ruled out, all treatments for your COPD, including lung transplant, as well as other surgery or procedures?
* Are you on solid, maximum treatment for COPD; best practice medications, and oxygen, if your tests indicate you need it?
* Have you discussed taking medications such as prednisone that help you breathe better, even if they might have some unwanted long-term side effects?
* Do you exercise regularly, even if it's very slow and minimal?
* Do you have a support group; family, friends, and other lung patients who understand what you're going through?
* Do you find it difficult to feel happy anymore?
* Have you had tests or screening to rule out any other major problems, such as heart disease?

If you answer yes to each of these questions, you've done all you can to keep on going, every step is a struggle, nothing relieves your shortness of breath, and you no longer feel joy in life – it's a good time to talk about this with your doctor.

So, what if this is "it?" A few thoughts on dying with COPD:

Hospice Care

First of all, it's important to understand that calling Hospice doesn't mean you have one foot in the grave and the other on a banana peel! It's all right to be in Hospice, even when you're still active! In fact, sometimes it even can allow you to be more active than you've recently been. Pulmonary rehab patients can be enrolled in Hospice and still come to maintenance (self-pay) exercise class.

Being in hospice takes pressure off of you about wondering how you're doing, and if you're doing the right things; and it takes a lot of stress off your loved ones. It bears repeating, it is all right to call hospice. And just think of it this way – if you talk with the people from hospice and they say you don't qualify, wouldn't that be good news?

Put it in writing

Complete your advance directive. There are two parts to this: Designation of an advocate who would speak for you if you were ever unable to speak for yourself; and a living will outlining the care and treatment you want and the care and treatment you don't want. Everyone should have an advance directive, even if you're young and healthy. For more on Advance Directives, see chapter October – Week 1.

Share your story

Everyone has a story to tell, and we should all pass ours along, whatever our age – or our health status. Make plans for a friend or a grandchild to listen as you tell your story; record it on audio, video, or digitally. Just sit down and start talking. You'll be so glad you did! Then, someday, even after you're gone, your words – and your spirit – will live on.

Be together

Make sure your family understands that when death is near, although a loved one might seem to be "out of it," or unconscious, very often they can still hear. A dying person can hear who is in the room, the news of the day – "Grandpa, I hit a home run today!" or "Dad, it's me, Mary. I'm here." – and most importantly, those precious "I love you's" right up to the end.

Give permission

If you're the loved one of a person with COPD and you see that he or she is suffering, give that person permission to die. Tell them that although you'll surely miss them, you will be able to go on without them and you'll be okay. People who are deathly ill often hang on and on, for fear that their loved one(s) will not be all right without them.

Treatment

Some medications that relieve pain and anxiety are also respiratory depressants, and doctors hesitate to prescribe them for people with COPD. Discuss this with your doctor and your hospice nurse, keeping in mind that *care and comfort is the goal*. The person who is dying – of any illness or disease – has the right to be as pain free and comfortable as possible.

Your Turn

Key points, or... If you don't remember anything else from this chapter, remember this:

- Dying is a part of life – for every one of us.
- Dying with COPD is all about your personal dignity and having your wishes (not someone else's) carried out in your final days.
- Make your wishes known by telling loved ones what you want. Then put it into writing.

Ask yourself this:

- Have I given thought to my passing, and talked with my loved ones about it?
- Do I have an Advance Directive? (See Chapter October – Week 1)

This week:

- If you answered "no" to the question about an Advance Directive, start to think about this and set up a time to talk with your doctor, a close family member or friend, or both.
- Consider sharing your story using the suggestions above.

Here's more help

- *The Grace in Dying,* by Kathleen Dowling Singh.

- *Final Gifts: Understanding the Special Awareness, Needs and Communications of the Dying,* by Maggie Callanan.
- GrowthHouse.org. Improving care for the dying http://www.growthhouse.org/

Your Most Commonly Asked Questions about Oxygen

Answered by Expert Lung Professionals
Francis Adams, MD; Robert Sandhaus, MD, PhD, FCCP
Helen Sorenson, MA, RRT, CPFT, FAARC

Experience tells you what to do;
confidence allows you to do it.
– Stan Smith

At BreathingBetterLivingWell.com we looked at hundreds of anonymous oxygen search questions (how people search for oxygen information on the Internet), and identified the ten most common. We then asked these questions of top lung professionals. Below are their answers. Thank-you to our BBLW Contributing Professionals for making the time to answer these important questions!

Please note: The responses below are not intended as medical advice but are for information only. Discuss this Q & A with your personal physician so he or she can advise you appropriately for your individual situation.

The first three questions were answered by Dr. Francis Adams.

1. What is a normal blood oxygen level?

Oxygen levels are commonly measured by two techniques. The first is a blood gas in which a blood sample is taken directly from an artery. This is the most accurate assessment of oxygen. The normal oxygen level using this technique is 80-100 (mmHg).

The second technique is bloodless and called pulse oximetry. The result here is not a direct measurement of oxygen but rather represents the percentage of hemoglobin that is saturated with oxygen. Hemoglobin is a protein in the blood that carries oxygen to the tissues. A light sensor is used which is commonly placed on a fingertip. Pulse oximetry is not as accurate as a blood gas and can be influenced by temperature and circulation. The normal oxygen saturation is 95%–100%.

2. Can I get addicted to oxygen?

I do not believe that you can become addicted to oxygen in the sense that one becomes compelled to use it as in alcoholism or heroin addiction. Many patients do become oxygen "dependent" because their bodies are unable to function without the use of oxygen supplementation. Oxygen is life sustaining and its use has prolonged life and improved its quality in individuals with inadequate levels.

3. How do I know when I need oxygen?

The most common symptom of a need for oxygen would be shortness of breath. When oxygen levels fall in the blood, nerve receptors in the neck recognize the deficiency and send distress signals to the brain. The result is the sensation of shortness of breath and an increase in the number of respirations per minute (rapid breathing). When oxygen levels are low a bluish hue might be noticed at the lips or fingertips, which is called cyanosis. Any patient experiencing shortness of breath should have an oxygen measurement.

The next three questions were answered by Dr. Robert Sandhaus.

4. Can too much oxygen hurt me?

There are some very specific situations in which it can be harmful to be on too much oxygen. However, for most people with COPD who receive oxygen through a nasal cannula, the answer is no, too much oxygen won't hurt you. Using too much oxygen is wasteful and can cause dryness and other discomforts.

So what are the situations in which too much oxygen can be harmful?

The brain regulates breathing based on the amount of carbon dioxide in the blood. Some individuals with very severe COPD retain carbon dioxide in their blood and the brain then begins to regulate breathing based on the amount of oxygen in the blood. Giving such a person too much oxygen can actually turn off their drive to breathe and cause life threatening respiratory arrest. Therefore, people with very severe COPD should check with their healthcare provider about whether they are at risk for this type of reaction to too much oxygen.

There are two other situations in which too much oxygen can be harmful. The first is giving high flow oxygen to newborn babies, which can cause blindness. The second is giving 100% oxygen to someone for a very long time, usually through a tube into the windpipe attached to a breathing machine or ventilator. Receiving very high amounts of oxygen over many days in this manner can injure lung cells.

5. Can too little oxygen hurt me?

If you need supplemental oxygen, not getting enough oxygen to raise your blood levels of oxygen to an appropriate level can have very serious long term effects. Too little oxygen causes the blood vessels in the lungs to constrict making it more difficult for the heart to pump blood through the lungs.

As a result, the pressure in the blood vessels feeding the lungs can rise, a condition known as Pulmonary Hypertension. If this goes on long enough the right side of the heart, the side that sends blood to the lungs, can fail, giving you a condition called right-sided heart failure, or Cor Pulmonale. In addition, if you don't have sufficient oxygen delivered to the tissues of the body, they can't function as they should. The organs most affected by low oxygen, in addition to the heart, are the muscles and the brain.

6. If I use my oxygen during the night when I sleep, can it carry over into the day?

The oxygen that gets into your blood by using supplemental oxygen leaves your system within several minutes after removing your cannula. Therefore, although the oxygen you use during the night can have many long-term beneficial effects, the oxygen itself is gone from your system fairly soon after you turn off the oxygen tank or concentrator. Many patients only need oxygen when they sleep and their oxygen levels are fine without supplemental oxygen during the day. But if you need oxygen both at night and during the day, using it only at night, while better than not using oxygen at all, is not sufficient to keep you well oxygenated during the day.

The last four questions were answered by Respiratory Therapist, Helen Sorenson.

7. I can't breathe, but my oxygen levels are normal.

8. I am on oxygen, but I am not breathing any better.

These are common questions and ones we hear all the time. Questions #7 and #8 are basically the same.

Dyspnea, or the sensation of difficult breathing, does not always correlate well with the amount of oxygen (O_2) in the blood. In other words, oxygen levels may be fine, but breathing is hard. When O_2 levels are okay and you may feel like you "can't breathe," your dyspnea is likely caused by anxiety often caused by the feeling of not being able to breathe. This can become a vicious cycle.

This is where pursed-lip breathing is most useful, because it slows down breathing, relaxes you, and often makes breathing easier. Another hint to decrease the sensation of difficult breathing is to sit in front of a fan – cool air facial stimulation decreases the sensation of dyspnea. Pulmonary rehabilitation patients tell me time and time again that the most important thing they learn from rehab is how to breathe correctly.

JMM – When the mechanics of breathing have been altered by over expanded lungs and a flattened diaphragm (the main muscle of breathing), it takes more work to move air in and out of your lungs. This added *work of breathing* causes shortness of breath. The oxygen exchange is still taking place, so you may have normal O_2 levels, but you still feel short of breath because your lungs and chest muscles are inefficient.

9. Can oxygen in my nose get in even when I have clogged sinuses?

That depends on the degree of obstruction/sinus congestion. If the nasal passages are completely swollen /

blocked, a cannula might not be as effective. But if your sinuses are congested just a little, you are likely breathing more through your mouth; then the oxygen going into the nasal passages will be pulled into the lungs by the air coming in through the mouth. I have seen patients put their cannula in their mouth, but that does not usually make the delivery of oxygen to the lungs any more effective.

10. At home, how long can my oxygen tubing be before the oxygen reaching me becomes less effective?

The length of the oxygen tubing should not affect the liter flow of oxygen being delivered. It just may take a little longer for the oxygen to get to you initially – like when it is first turned on – but once it is flowing, it should remain constant.

Even though oxygen is a gas, we should think of it in terms of being a liquid – if the pressure at the tank remains constant (which it does until the tank has less than 500 psi), the liter flow, 2 LPM (liters per minute), 3 LPM, etc. will remain constant. Think in terms of a garden hose – if the pressure/flow of water coming out of the faucet is constant, regardless of the length of the hose, the same amount of water will exit the other end. The only thing that may affect oxygen delivery is if there is an occlusion/obstruction in the tubing.

Your Turn

Key points, or ... If you don't remember anything else from this chapter, remember this:

- We all need oxygen, and have, since the moment we were born.

- If tests show that you require supplemental oxygen, you should use it as prescribed.
- Using oxygen as directed will help prolong your life and take stress off your other major body systems.

Ask yourself this:

- Am I doing all I can to use my oxygen as prescribed?
- Have I checked with my oxygen provider to make sure the system I'm using is the best for me and my lifestyle?

This week:

- If you don't already have a home pulse oximeter, talk with your doctor about getting one for use at home.

Here's more help

- *Adventures of an Oxy-Phile2*, by Thomas Petty, MD.
- Information about getting around with oxygen http://www.portableoxygen.org/overview.html

Lung Disease: Unseen and Misunderstood
[JVT/JMM]

Sick lungs don't show.
– John W. Walsh

"Which one of us is going to limp today?" said Mary Pierce to her husband Todd, as they got out of their car and walked towards the entrance of the store. They were used to getting dirty looks as they parked in the handicapped parking spot.

"People watched us getting out of the car and you just knew what they were thinking. They didn't see either of us with crutches – or a wheel chair. They didn't see my lungs, how bad they were, especially because I was young, like many of the Alphas." (Alpha-1 Antitrypsin Deficiency is a genetically inherited form of COPD that manifests in people as early as in their teens and twenties. See Chapter April – Week 1.)

One of the most difficult aspects of dealing with chronic lung disease is that it is rarely understood by those who are not personally affected by it. Close family members and / or spouses may eventually learn a good bit about the devastating effects of COPD, lung cancer, bronchiectasis, Alpha-1 Antitrypsin Deficiency, cystic fibrosis, pulmonary fibrosis, or other specific diseases of the pulmonary and respiratory systems. But sadly, some never do.

Having pulmonary disease can cause disabilities that, while enormously restricting and progressively debilitating, are not obvious to a casual observer. That extends also to friends, employers, and neighbors. All around us we find people who don't understand that there are certain things we simply can no longer physically do for ourselves. Nor do they comprehend what a price we pay for having to ask for help, or how it erodes our self-esteem.

All of us wish to maintain as much of the personal pride and dignity we can. So, what can we, as patients, do to help others understand? In my experience, education about pulmonary disease is the key to improved emotional support from our friends and loved ones. We need to take it upon ourselves, as a mission, to bring every opportunity to learn about lung disease to those around us, even to the general public.

As we learn more ourselves, we should look for ways to get that vital information to spouses, relatives, even our friends and neighbors. Help them know the symptoms of this disease, the restrictions, and what it takes to fight our way to maintain stability or to improve from an exacerbation. But, we must make sure we do this with a positive attitude, reminding them of what we still can do.

We have to encourage our spouses or caregivers to join us at support group meetings, where they can listen and learn from guest speakers, or from the patients themselves. Siblings are also welcome at meetings, as well as our sons and daughters.

The most important thing to remember is this: We should invest our energy in positive things that we can do for ourselves, and then we'll be better able to do whatever we can to have a deeper understanding of this disease, for ourselves and others. This will go a long way toward achieving our goal of holding onto as much quality of life as possible, and also bring lung disease out of the shadows.

Your Turn

Key points, or ... If you don't remember anything else from this chapter, remember this:

- Most of the time, lung disease cannot be seen by others, making it difficult for them to understand it.
- It is up to you to help educate those close to you about your lung disease; how it limits your ability to function, but also about thing you are able to do.

Ask yourself this:

- Have you explained to those you care about what COPD is and how it affects you?

This week:

- Invite a close friend or family member to come with you to your next support group meeting, or show them a website and / or online forum for people with COPD.

Here's more help

- But You Don't Look Sick
  http://www.butyoudontlooksick.com
- Breathing Better, Living Well community forum
  http://www.breathingbetterlivingwell.com/community/index.php

- American Lung Association – Find a Better
  Breathers Club in Your Area
  Phone: 800-586-4872
  http://www.lungusa.org/lung-disease/copd/
  connect-with-others/better-breathers-clubs/

Learning to Breathe Again
Part I – Pursed-Lip Breathing
[JMM]

Learn something new each day.
– Iris Carlyle

You'd think that breathing would be as easy as inhaling and exhaling, something you wouldn't have to think about at all. But as a person with COPD, you know that sometimes staying in control of your breathing can be very difficult – in fact, almost impossible. This week we're going to talk about proper breathing techniques with COPD. *As always, check with your doctor or respiratory health care professional before starting any new technique or exercise.*

Why are we even talking about *learning* how to breathe? You might be thinking, "I've been breathing since the moment I was born so why – and how – am I suddenly supposed to *learn* how to breathe?" The answer is simple. If you have COPD, there have been changes in your lungs and possibly, your chest, that keep you from being able to breathe as nature intended. In order to understand proper breathing techniques and how to use them effectively, you first need to know what's going on in your lungs.

COPD is a combination of emphysema and chronic bronchitis. When you have COPD, especially with a significant component of emphysema, your lungs are hyper-inflated – stretched out and filled with too much stale air. So, your lungs are actually too big; they're crowded inside your chest and don't have a lot of room to move. To breathe with over-inflated lungs can take a whole lot of work with not a whole lot of results. This is one of the main reasons why breathing with COPD can be so difficult.

Also in COPD, the inside walls of your airways (the tubes inside your lungs that the air travels through) can become weak and collapse. I don't have to tell you that if your airways collapse, that's a problem that can make breathing even harder.

There are two main breathing techniques that help when you have COPD. Each of these techniques works to compensate for specific things that have gone wrong with the mechanics of breathing brought on by COPD. One method is Pursed-Lips Breathing (PLB) and the other is Diaphragmatic Breathing (DB), also called abdominal or belly breathing. This week we're going to talk about Pursed-Lips Breathing.

Let's review the problems and then talk about how PLB helps.

Problem:
Weak airway walls make it more likely for airways to collapse, preventing the air from getting out. When you huff and puff, you breathe out too hard and this can collapse weak airways.
Solution:
With PLB done correctly you create "back pressure" on the inside walls of the airways, holding the airways open.

Problem:
Over inflation of the lungs causes air-trapping. The lungs become stretched out, lose their elasticity, and become crowded inside the chest.

Solution:

Using proper PLB helps you expel more of the stale, trapped air. By doing this, you can't return your lungs to a normal size, but you can help slow down the rate of even more air trapping.

Problem:

Carbon dioxide (CO_2), the waste product of breathing sometimes builds up because there is too much trapped air inside your lungs. Retaining too much CO_2 can throw off your essential acid / base balance and affect other body systems.

Solution:

Exhaling for a longer period of time with correct PLB can rid your lungs of more CO_2.

Problem:

Huffing and puffing with exertion is exhausting and frustrating, and can lead to feelings of anxiety, even panic.

Solution:

Proper PLB allows a person with COPD to have greater endurance and activity tolerance and also have a feeling of being calm and in control.

Disclaimer: This information is not to be substituted for medical advice. Always consult your doctor before starting any new exercise or technique. These breathing techniques should be demonstrated and taught by a pulmonary health care professional, and when beginning, should be practiced by the patient for a few minutes at a time, a few times a day. Feel free to bring this information to your doctor and ask him or her if working with these breathing retraining techniques would be appropriate for you.

What is Pursed-Lips Breathing (PLB), and how is it done?

PLB is the first line of defense used by most COPDers when trying to recover from, or avoid, shortness of breath. It involves breathing in through the nose and exhaling with the lips pursed, as if you are going to whistle. How hard do you blow out? It's simple. Blow out with the same force that you would use to cool hot soup on a spoon. Blow hard enough to cool it, but not hard enough to blow it off the spoon.

Here is a start on learning Pursed-Lips Breathing

Begin by relaxing your shoulders, and while still sitting up straight, let your shoulders fall as low as possible. For people with COPD, it is common to have a lot of upper body tension. You will not be able to do breathing retraining effectively if your shoulders are elevated and tense.

Pursed-Lips Breathing

1. Inhale slowly through your nose.
2. Purse your lips, or pucker them gently, as if you are going to whistle.
3. Breathe out slowly while keeping your lips pursed.
4. Take twice as long to breathe out as you do to breathe in. For example, if you breathe in for a count of two seconds, breathe out for four seconds.

5. Never force your air out. Just let it flow out
through your pursed lips.
Pursed-lip breathing will help you:
* Slow down your breathing
* Get rid of more of the stale, trapped air, and car-
bon dioxide (CO_2).
* Be in control of your breathing, instead of your
breathing controlling you!

If done properly, using the right breathing techniques
will go a long way in helping you move more air and stay
in control your breathing.

Your Turn

**Key points, or . . . If you don't remember anything else
from this chapter, remember this:**

- Pursed-lips breathing can help you control your
breathing instead of letting your breathing take
over and control you.
- Never hold your breath!
- Keep your shoulders down and as relaxed as
possible.
- Use PLB whenever you exert yourself.
- If you work on PLB regularly, it will eventually
come naturally without having to think about it.

Ask yourself this:

- When I'm short of breath, am I able to gain control over my breathing with PLB?

This week:

- If PLB is new to you, or if you don't use it regularly, ask your doctor if it is all right for you to

try. If so, practice it for a few minutes, five to ten times each day.

Here's more help

- Based on the article "Pursed-Lip Breathing: Pucker Up and Breathe Easier," by Jane M. Martin, BA,LRT,CRT, and published on COPDConnection.com. Copyright 2008, HealthCentral. All rights reserved. http://www.healthcentral.com/copd/c/19257/18835/lip-breathing-breathe
- "Diaphragmatic and Pursed Lip Breathing" by Dr Vijai Sharma
- MindPub.com http://www.mindpub.com/art574.htm
- *Anatomy of Breathing*, by Blandine Calais-Germain

Learning to Breathe Again
Part II – Diaphragmatic Breathing
[JMM]

When somebody says to me – which they do, like, every
five years – 'How does it feel to be over the hill?'
My response is, 'I'm just heading up the mountain.'
– Joan Baez

I hope you've read the July – Week 1 chapter about Pursed-Lips Breathing. If you haven't, please do, because although these two breathing techniques can be done independently you'll receive the most benefit if you learn them together. As always, check with your doctor or respiratory health care professional before starting any new technique or exercise.

If you have COPD, Diaphragmatic Breathing (DB) is another important breathing technique to learn. It is also called belly, or abdominal, breathing. Doing diaphragmatic breathing (and doing it correctly) can mean the difference between huffing and puffing and struggling your way through each day, or being in control of your breathing as you do the things you want, and need, to do.

First of all, let's review why we're even talking about learning how to breathe. Again, you may be thinking, "I've been breathing since the moment I was born so why am I suddenly supposed to 'learn' how to breathe?" The answer is simple. If you have COPD there have been changes in your lungs and possibly, in your chest, that have caused changes to the way you were born to breathe.

So, what's going on in my lungs? Some of this material is a review from chapter March – Week 4, but it relates closely with lung anatomy and physiology, as well as proper breathing techniques.

When lungs become damaged from cigarette smoking or other hazards in the environment, the elastic fibers within them start to deteriorate and the lungs begin to lose their elastic recoil – their ability to *get air out* effectively. You can think of this by comparing a balloon to a paper bag. The air in the balloon comes out easily because the balloon is elastic and expels the air as it deflates. A paper bag is not. Over the years the loss of your lungs' elastic recoil gets worse and the lungs develop *air trapping and over-inflation.*

This means that your lungs actually become bigger than they should be. And this leads to trouble, because the excess stale air compresses functioning lung tissue so it can't do the job it should – kind of like when the air bag in your car inflates and is pressing on your chest. When your lungs are too big for the inside of your chest, it's crowded in there and your lungs have trouble expanding and recoiling. Also, when this happens, your diaphragm, which is supposed to be in the shape of a dome, becomes flatter, putting you – and your lung movement – at a mechanical disadvantage.

When the natural function of lung movement is less effective, you automatically begin to recruit the muscles around your collarbone, your neck, and between your ribs to move your lungs. Using these muscles to breathe not only takes a lot of energy but it can make you sore and tense in your shoulders and your back. In addition to this, you're not using that most efficient muscle of breathing, the strongest breathing muscle you have, your diaphragm, to do most of the work. More work of breathing combined with less efficient lung movement adds up to a whole lot of effort and fatigue without a lot of results!

Problem:
The diaphragm becomes flattened at rest. It works best when it is in a dome-shape at rest.
Solution:
Diaphragmatic breathing can help strengthen that muscle to work more effectively even though it's at a mechanical disadvantage.

Problem:
Rapid, shallow breathing.
Solution:
Proper diaphragmatic breathing is slower, deeper breathing.

Problem:
Increased use of accessory breathing muscles.
Solution:
Better use of the diaphragm lessens the need to use inefficient accessory muscles.

Diaphragmatic (Belly or Abdominal) Breathing

Your diaphragm is a large, flat sheet of muscle just below your lungs and above your abdomen (your belly). It was meant to do most of the work of breathing, but people with COPD tend to huff and puff, causing them to use the weaker muscles around the collarbone and between the ribs. By using your diaphragm when you breathe, you help your lungs expand more fully so they take in more air with less effort.

When the diaphragm flattens, pulling on the bottoms of your lungs, your belly – your abdomen – should extend. Yes, just like your tummy is looking bigger. When you breathe out properly, the diaphragm should go up, pushing on the bottoms of your lungs, helping you get rid of the stale, trapped air.

Disclaimer: This information is not to be substituted for medical advice. Always consult your doctor before starting any new exercise or technique. These breathing techniques should be demonstrated and taught by a pulmonary health care professional, and when beginning, should be practiced for a just a few minutes at a time, a few times a day. Show this information to your doctor and ask him or her if doing these breathing techniques would be appropriate for you.

Diaphragmatic breathing can be a difficult concept to understand and a tough technique to master. It takes practice, but it's worth it! Below are the basic steps. Learning it works best in a reclining position.

1. Relax your shoulders. Drop them down as low as they'll go.
2. Put your hands on your abdomen with your fingers overlapped, but not intertwined, just below your ribs.
3. Breathe in slowly through your nose, making your abdomen push out while you breathe in. (Remember to keep those shoulders down!)
4. Breathe out slowly, about twice as long as you breathed in, using pursed lips. Gently, with your hands, push your belly in and think about expelling all that stale air.

5. Practice this from time to time throughout the day for a few minutes at a time.

If you experience muscle soreness or fatigue with this technique it is probably because you are either working too hard at it or not doing it correctly. That's why you should learn this technique only with the supervision of a person who specializes in proper breathing techniques. Once you catch on, you should be able to breathe easier and be less tired. Using this technique, along with pursed-lips breathing, will go a long way in helping you exert more, with less shortness of breath, and also help you work through anxious episodes.

One more word of caution – be careful of breathing methods or devices you may read about in magazines or see on the Internet. Remember, if something sounds too good to be true, it probably is! Before you spend your money on any breathing aid not ordered by your doctor, check with your doctor or a respiratory health professional.

Using proper breathing techniques with COPD can mean the difference between struggling to get through your day – or being in control and breathing easier.

Your Turn

Key points, or . . . If you don't remember anything else from this chapter, remember this:

- Changes in your lungs lead to inefficient breathing patterns just when you have less energy and oxygen available.
- Doing diaphragmatic breathing can mean the difference between huffing and puffing or being in control of your breathing.

Ask yourself this:

- What breathing muscles am I using the most to help my air go in and out?

This week:

- If diaphragmatic breathing (DB) is new to you, or if you don't use it regularly, practice it for a few minutes, five times each day. DB is more difficult to master than PLB, so if you become tired or frustrated, just give yourself a break and try again later.

Here's more help

- Here's a simple animation that shows how the diaphragm works. http://www.nlhep.org/lung_intro.html
- *The Breathing Book: Vitality & Good Health Through Essential Breath Work,* by Donna Farhi

Relaxation
[Vijai Sharma, PhD]

A field that has rested gives a bountiful crop.
– Ovid

Disclaimer: This information is not to be substituted for medical advice. Always consult your doctor before starting any new exercise or technique. Show this information to your doctor and ask him or her if doing these relaxation techniques would be appropriate for you.

People mean different things by the word "relax." For some, relaxing means coming home from work, taking their shoes off, sipping a drink, reading the paper, or watching TV; while for others, relaxation is that nap they sneak in during the day. Some people find it relaxing to go for a run. Moments of quietude, without being angry and upset, is relaxation for others.

Actually, physical and mental relaxation means undoing the physical and mental stress or tension you are experiencing at the time. There are people who are apprehensive of the word relaxation, viewing it with suspicion and hesitancy. They fear that if they begin to relax, they will become lazy, unproductive, and lose the "fight" in them. Nothing could be further from the truth. Relaxation can nourish you, make you stronger, and help you be better prepared to fight any challenge you might face.

We do not always recognize that we are tense even when we are, and this is especially true if you have COPD. Most people who are habitually tense have been that way for many years. Tension and stress have become the natural state of their body and mind. They are unaware of the tension they carry with them day and night, twenty-four hours a day, seven days a week. If they were asked, "Are you tense?" They would respond, "No! I'm okay," because they have not truly experienced relaxation and thus do not know the difference.

Benefits of Relaxation

I often wonder, with so many effective relaxation methods available today, why people are attracted to sleeping pills and chemical relaxants. Relaxation techniques can help us to sleep and feel better, naturally. The effects of sleeping pills and chemical relaxants wear off over time, as one develops a tolerance for them.

With relaxation techniques, the more you use them, the more effective they become. When you can deepen your relaxation, you can enjoy it even more. And unlike sleeping pills or other chemical relaxants, there are no bad side effects of relaxation techniques! Regular practice of mental and physical relaxation may help you, also, to breathe more easily and may relieve part of your breathing discomfort.

It takes about fifteen to twenty minutes to complete a full relaxation session. In the beginning, it is more effective to learn relaxation by using full relaxation methods. If your stress level, pain, or another type of challenge is really high, do two or three full sessions a day. One session a day is good, two times better, and three times is excellent.

Once basic relaxation skills are acquired, you will be able to relax quickly and easily, without taking so much time. Practice full and short methods frequently. Quick methods take the wind out of the sails of the stress ship. When you are actually in the middle of a challenging situation, you can apply quick methods right then and there, in the face of the situation.

Record and Play

You may record the scripts of the relaxation sessions in your own voice and play them during your relaxation session. After sufficient practice these words will become part of you and you won't need to play them.

Full Relaxation Method (15-20 minutes)

Preparation for Relaxation

Relaxation exercise can be performed lying or sitting down. If you prefer to lie down, make sure you have proper pillow support under your neck and lower back or knees, if needed. Lie if you prefer, or sit, making yourself comfortable. Sit with arms and hands in the lap or the thighs; back, neck and head straight but relaxed.

Affirmation

Silently or aloud say to yourself with conviction, "I will do my best to relax physically and mentally in spite of annoying problems such as outside noise, cough, shortness of breath, or pain. Thoughts, feelings, and sensations may interrupt me but I can quickly bring my mind to the part of the body I want to relax. Staying relaxed and calm, I simply bring my attention to each part of the body."

Begin

* Feet relax...Relaxing soles of my feet, toes and ankle joints...
* Legs from ankle joints to knee joints...
* From knee joints to thigh joints.
* Relaxing, pelvis...abdomen...midsection...and chest.
* Relaxing, my hips...lower back...mid-back...and upper back.
* My whole upper body relaxes...front...back...from inside...from outside...my entire upper body relaxes.
* Ahhh! (Sigh while exhaling.)
* Relaxing shoulders, shoulder pads, and the shoulder blades...now the space between the shoulder blades.
* Relaxing my upper arms from shoulder joints to elbow joints...
* Upper arms and elbows, lower down toward the hips...
* Forearms to wrists...
* Hands, relax all the way down to my fingertips.
* The top of my hands and palms relax.
* Nice, lazy, relaxing feeling of warmth and heaviness...
* From fingertips all the way up through my arms and shoulders...
* The back of my neck and head relaxes.
* All the tiny and large muscles in my neck and throat relax.
* Feeling of relaxation spreads over to the nape of the neck...back of the head...over my entire scalp...down to my forehead.

* Forehead feels smooth, like the touch of lavender or a cool breeze.
* The feeling of relaxation flows down my face.
* Nostrils relax and feel more open than before.
* Any blockages in the upper part of my nose relax and shrink.
* Sinuses relax and open up.
* My jaw relaxes.
* Gums, teeth, tongue, hard and soft palate, and the throat, relax from inside.
* I observe my breathing without trying to change it in any way.
* While inhaling through my nose, silently saying, "In 1-2."
* While exhaling through pursed lips, silently saying, "Out 1-2-3-4."
* "In 1-2…Out 1-2-3-4."
* "In 1-2…Out 1-2-3-4."
* "In 1-2…Out 1-2-3-4."
* "In 1-2…Out 1-2-3-4."
* "In 1-2…Out 1-2-3-4."

* I imagine I'm breathing in as if through the crown of my head and breathing out through the toes and the soles of my feet.
* "In 1-2…Out 1-2-3-4."
* "In 1-2…Out 1-2-3-4."
* "In 1-2…Out 1-2-3-4."
* "In 1-2…Out 1-2-3-4."
* "In 1-2…Out 1-2-3-4."

* My neck and shoulders become more relaxed and loose.

* Shoulders are back and down...shoulder blades slightly lowered towards the mid-back.
* Diaphragm is soft, relaxed, and increased in length. It contracts and relaxes as I breathe.
* When I exhale, my diaphragm goes up higher than ever before and pushes up against the bottom of my lungs, expelling the air more completely.
* I picture my diaphragm attached to my lower ribs as a sheath, separating my abdomen from my lower chest.
* As my diaphragm moves, the lower ribs also move. Muscles between my ribs are becoming strong and flexible, helping my ribcage to move.
* I exhale softly and slowly. My diaphragm on both sides goes up like a dome, pushing at the bottom of my lungs.
* The center of the diaphragm goes up and massages my heart at the same time.
* As the diaphragm moves up, lower ribs drop slightly lower, down toward the hips.
* I exhale and feel the diaphragm moving up towards the lungs.
* As I breathe in softly and gently, my diaphragm goes down...side ribs spread out and up, like wings on both sides.
* My ribcage lifts, lumbar curve arches...at the same time, my abdomen between the navel and the breastbone tip, lengthens.

Visualization

Picture for a few minutes in your "mind's eye" any of the following: The place you would like to be right now or the time of your life you loved and enjoyed most. Spend as much time as you have. Savor that time and place in your mind.

Short Relaxation 5-10 minutes

Preparation for Relaxation

Relaxation exercise can be done lying or sitting down. If you prefer to lie down, make sure you have proper pillow support under your neck and lower back or knees, if needed. Lie if you prefer, or sit, making yourself comfortable. Sit with arms and hands in the lap or the thighs; back, neck and head straight but relaxed.

Affirmation

* Silently or aloud say to yourself with conviction, "I will do my best to relax physically and mentally in spite of annoying problems such as outside noise, cough, shortness of breath, or pain. Thoughts, feelings, and sensations may interrupt me but I can quickly bring my mind to the part of the body I want to relax. Staying relaxed and calm, I simply bring my attention to each part of the body."
* Relaxing shoulders, shoulder pads, and the shoulder blades...now the space between the shoulder blades.
* Relaxing the upper arms from shoulder joints to elbow joints...
* Upper arms and elbows, lower down to forearms to wrists...
* Hands relax all the way down to the fingertips.
* The top of my hands and palms relax.
* Nice, lazy, relaxing feeling of warmth and heaviness...

* From fingertips all the way up through the arms and shoulders…
* The back of my neck and head relaxes.
* All the tiny and large muscles in my neck and throat relax.
* Feeling of relaxation spreads over to the nape of the neck…back of the head…over the entire scalp…down to my forehead.
* Forehead feels smooth, like the touch of lavender or a cool breeze.
* The feeling of relaxation flows down my face.
* Nostrils relax and feel more open than before.
* Any blockages in the upper part of my nose relax and shrink.
* Sinuses relax and open up.
* My jaw relaxes.

* While inhaling, silently saying, "In…1-2."
* While exhaling, silently saying, "Out…1-2-3-4."
* "In 1-2…Out 1-2-3-4."
* "In 1-2…Out 1-2-3-4."
* "In 1-2…Out 1-2-3-4."
* "In 1-2…Out 1-2-3-4."
* "In 1-2…Out 1-2-3-4."
* "In 1-2…Out 1-2-3-4."
* "In 1-2…Out 1-2-3-4."
* "In 1-2…Out 1-2-3-4."
* "In 1-2…Out 1-2-3-4."
* "In 1-2…Out 1-2-3-4."

Your Turn

Key points, or…If you don't remember anything else from this chapter, remember this:

- It is important for us to relax, especially with COPD.
- You are probably tense, possibly very tense, and don't even realize it.
- Anyone can learn relaxation techniques.
- Relaxation techniques, once learned, can help you feel better and breathe better.

Ask yourself this:

- When is the last time I felt truly relaxed?

This week:

- Take fifteen to twenty minutes each day to go to a quiet place and work on the full relaxation session.

Here's more help

- http://www.mindpub.com
- Excerpted from the book *Overcoming Anxiety and Depression – Breathing Correctly in COPD/ Emphysema: A Self Care Book for People with COPD and a Psychosocial Manual for Professionals,* by Vijai Sharma, PhD, intended for future publication. Copyright©2008, Vijai Sharma,PhD. (all inquiries to be directed to dr.sharma@mindpub.com)
- *800 Stepping Stones to Complete Relaxation: Physical, Emotional, Sleep, Dream, Mental, Creativity, Self, Visualization, Projection,* by Michael Lee Wright

Keeping a Journal
[JVT]

*I can't write a book commensurate with Shakespeare
but I can write a book by me.*
– Sir Water Raleigh

For a long time, I've extolled the virtues of keeping a journal, and have tried to encourage people in our support group to write about their experiences with lung disease. It's mentioned frequently in my book on COPD, *Courage and Information for Life with Chronic Obstructive Lung Disease*; in fact, that's how the book began. After a while, writing in my journal prompted me to think about turning it into a manuscript, in order to provide help to others through my own perspectives as a COPD patient.

You might think that writing is only for people who are good spellers or are especially articulate, but here's a good example why keeping a journal is beneficial for almost anyone. And we now know that it is especially helpful to those with a chronic disease.

Some time ago a study on journaling was done at the State University of New York at Stony Brook. A report on this study that appeared in the journal of the American Medical Association said, "Writing about traumatic life experiences helps patients suffering from asthma or rheumatoid arthritis improve their health."

Here's how the study was done: Researcher Joshua Smyth and colleagues in Stony Brook's psychiatry department separated a group of 112 asthma and arthritis patients and asked them to spend twenty minutes daily, over three days, writing either about their most stressful life events or about ordinary things, such as their daily schedule. Those with arthritis who wrote about their trauma reported a 28% reduction in disease severity within four months, while the control group showed no change. Asthmatics who wrote about their trauma showed a 19% increase in lung function against no change in the control group.

"We don't want to tell people to throw away their medicines," said Smyth... "But what this study tells us is that we need to pay attention to psychological factors when we are talking about the treatment of chronic illness."

.... Overall, an analysis of the findings showed that 47% of the patients who wrote about their trauma were reported by an independent physician to be clinically improved, compared to 24% of the control patients."

Please understand, as Mr. Smyth indicates, this is not to say, by any means, that keeping a journal should replace any of your medications or treatments. But, ask yourself, "With this information in mind, would it harm me to spend a few minutes each day writing?"

Do yourselves a favor, my friends. Invest a couple bucks in a notebook, or create a journal file in your computer, and invest your time in writing every day. The blank page will listen to what you have to say, and no one else need ever read it, unless you want them to. You can express your feelings, your frustrations, your fears and your triumphs – at your own pace, in your own way. Keep it in a private place, and allow this wonderful form of self-expression to capture the thoughts that can't easily be shared out loud. Twenty minutes of writing our thoughts in a journal each day is painless, harmful to no one, and is an inexpensive therapist.

When I attended the funeral service of a departed member of our Cape Cod COPD Support Group, I was particularly moved when one of his daughters read from the pages of his daily journal. She said he started writing the journal to document his struggles with COPD, and to mark the really good days so he could remember them on the bad days. I'm sure that it did not occur to this man that his words would bring comfort to his family and friends after he was gone. But they did.

Even the writing I do to produce this Newsletter has helped me personally, just as writing my book was cathartic for my soul. I suspect that together, these two projects are responsible for a lot of my COPD stability over the years, and for a significant lift in my spirit and my heart. Thank you for reading. I hope my writing efforts – labors of love, really – have brought and will continue to provide an equal share of comfort and healing to you, as well.

Bonus Box
Josie's experience with keeping a journal

I had never been in a hospital before except to have two babies, but I found myself there because of my breathing. I wondered, "What am I doing here all hooked up, everything imaginable going into me?" I was frightened. Who wouldn't be? After I was well again, I knew I had to do something new, so on the way home I thought, "Okay, let's give this a try."

I got a little book. Every day in the page on the left I recorded what medicines I took, how I felt, who came to visit me, what I did, whether I wrote checks – just little things. What did I do today? How many times did I take my inhaler? Was there something good on television? It seems so insignificant, I know.

But I can look back in my journal and see what exercises I was doing, and what exercises I actually am doing now. It keeps me on track. You'd be surprised how fast a year goes, and how interesting it is to look back and see what you were doing. I can go back just a year and see what I was doing each day. I was doing tai chi, walking three times, taking a nap, and I got one of those little stationary bicycles that you sit in the chair and wheel. I did that every day.

On the page on the right, I write down good things that happen. Happy things. Things I'm thankful for. I've been doing this, let's see….well, this is my fourth year.

I would encourage everyone to make a little diary. It might seem unimportant to you, but it works for me. Try it and it might work for you too!

Your Turn

Key points, or … If you don't remember anything else from this chapter, remember this:

- If you have COPD, writing in a journal each day can help you feel better.
- Writing in a journal is an easy, inexpensive way to help you stay focused and on track with caring for your COPD.

Ask yourself this:

- Am I willing to try keeping a simple journal this week?

This week:

- Get a lined tablet, no smaller than 5 x 7 inches. Each day write enough to fill at least half a page. You can write about your COPD – if you're having a good day, a bad day, if you went somewhere, if you exercised, or what you ate. Just write about whatever comes to mind. Make it a habit and see how you feel at the end of the week.

Here's more help

- For more information on the journaling study at Stony Brook, visit http://www.breathingbetterlivingwell.com/archive/articles/journwritngstudy.pdf.
- *One Journal's Life: A Meditation on Journal-Keeping,* by Audrey Borenstein
- "The Benefits of Journaling for Stress Management," by Elizabeth Scott, M.S.
- http://stress.about.com/od/generaltechniques/p/profilejournal.htm

Medications
[JMM]

Experience tells you what to do;
confidence allows you to do it.
– Stan Smith

Some time ago I was teaching a series of COPD and asthma management classes to home care nurses, explaining how important it is for pulmonary patients to understand their inhaled medications – how to take them for maximum benefit, how they differ from each other, and how each one is supposed to work.

A nurse told a story about one of her patients with COPD. She was about to end her visit for that day when from across the room she saw a very large ashtray (yes, an ashtray!) filled to overflowing with a variety of inhalers. She asked the patient about the use of these inhalers and he casually said, "Oh, when I feel tight I just take a couple puffs off this one or that one or another one until I start to feel better." Yikes! Not exactly what I'd call informed or effective use of inhaled pulmonary medication!

When I ask patients what their inhalers do, they almost always respond by saying simply, "They open up my lungs." Well, yes, that's true, but what's really important for all patients with COPD to know and understand is there are different types of medicines that open the airways in different ways.

This is kind of complicated but it is not all that difficult to understand, so put your thinking caps on, and grab a pencil to jot down notes if you need to. I suggest you make your marks in this book and circle the names of the medicines you're on and underline or highlight the categories they are in. This will help you understand what each breathing medicine is supposed to do. If you're borrowing this book, it's okay to make a copy of this chapter for your personal use and make notes on your copy.

Note: Although every effort was taken to make this chapter as complete and accurate as possible in late 2010, the lists as you find them here may not necessarily be all-inclusive, nor up to date, when you read them. Medications come and go, although many are in use for decades. This will, however, give you a pretty good understanding of what does what, and how, so you can understand your own medications and take them with maximum effectiveness.

Here we go. I'm going to start out by breaking things down into major categories and then we'll continue down the lists to learn more as we go along.

Fire Prevention and Calling 911

There are two different, very basic, ways that medicines act to open up the airways in your lungs: Prevention, with these being referred to as Maintenance or Controllers – and Rescue, referred to as Rescue or Relievers. For the sake of this discussion, let's use the words Prevention and Rescue and we'll refer to the medicines as either Preventers or Rescuers.

An easy way to understand Prevention and Rescue in breathing medicines is looking at the situation as we look at fire.

Prevention: As a responsible person, you do your best to prevent fires; for example, by maintaining your home, keeping the electrical wires operating safely, turning the stove off when you're not using it, and putting hot matches in a ceramic dish or in water. All these things prevent a fire from starting. If you skip any of these steps, what might happen? Well, you could have a raging blaze. And we all know it makes a lot more sense to prevent a fire than to allow one to start!

Rescue: If and when a fire does start, however, you have (or should have) a fire extinguisher handy. And we also have the 911 system to call for help. Thank goodness! But, again, if you can prevent a fire from starting – even knowing all the while that you have help to put it out – you should make the effort.

You can think of medicines for your lungs in much the same way. Use the prevention medications as directed to be as effective as possible, to keep your airways (bronchial tubes) inside your lungs from swelling up, causing spasms and getting tight. If, however, you do all you can to prevent this and you still run into problems, it's time to reach for your rescue medication.

Preventers

Inhaled medications that work as preventers come in three different types.

- ∗ Corticosteroids
- ∗ Anticholinergics
- ∗ Long-acting Bronchodilators (beta-2 agonists)

I know this is sounding kind of complicated, but stay with me here.

Corticosteroids work to reduce inflammation or swelling on the insides of your bronchial tubes. Think of it in this way: Ten of us can be in one room, breathing in the same air. Each of us may have a different reaction to what we breathe in. Some of us would be fine, but others might develop tight breathing because they happen to have bronchial tubes that are far more sensitive than others.

Likewise, ten of us could go to the beach on the same day. We might each of us experience a different reaction to the sun. Some of us might tan and some of us might burn. If you are the one who gets sunburned, would you think about going home from a day at the beach and putting on sunscreen? Of course not! That wouldn't make sense. You can think of corticosteroids as sunscreen for the insides of your sensitive bronchial airways. They are preventers. You should take them every day to keep your bronchial airways from becoming inflamed and swollen on the insides.

Coricosteroids are:
* Qvar
* Pulmicort
* Flovent
* Aerobid
* Asmanex
* Alvesco

Combination inhaled medicines with steroids are: (see also Combination Corticosteroids and Long-acting Bronchodilators)
* Advair (Flovent and Serevent)
* Symbicort (Foradil and Pulmicort)
* Dulera (Foradil and Asmanex)

The next category is **Anticholinergics**.

These medications work to block the message that causes spasms of smooth muscles in the airways of the lungs. So they actually stop airway muscle tightening before it starts, preventing it; kind of like putting a road-block in the way of something that can start a problem. Anticholinergics are:

* Atrovent
* Spiriva

Long-acting Bronchodilators is the third category of preventers.

These medicines work to relax the muscles around your airways (bronchial tubes) and prevent squeezing. Medicines that are in this long-acting category do not begin to work as soon as you take them; they take about twenty minutes. But, they last for about twelve hours. Therefore, if you take them twelve hours apart, you should have around the clock coverage for preventing those muscles from acting up and squeezing your airways.

Long-acting Bronchodilators are:

* Foradil
* Brovana
* Serevent
* Performist

Combination Corticosteroids and Long-Acting Bronchodilators

There are many folks who have COPD and asthma who benefit from both inhaled corticosteroids and a long-acting bronchodilator, so it makes sense to combine these two medications into one inhaler. Below are three such medications.

Combination Corticosteroids and Long-Acting Bronchodilators are:

* Advair – a combination of Flovent and Serevent
* Symbicort – a combination of Pulmicort and Foradil

* Dulera – a combination of Asmanex and Foradil

Rescuers

Short (fast)-acting Bronchodilators (Beta-2 agonists)

These medicines, like those above, work to relax the muscles around your airways (bronchial tubes) to prevent squeezing, but they go to work soon after you take them. This is good, but, they last for only about four to six hours (with the exception of Xopenex which works for twelve hours). Remember, our goal is to use these medicines as little as possible. This is because it's better to keep your airways open without giving them the chance to flare up. There is some research suggesting that repeated flare-ups over time, cause permanent lung damage.

Short-acting bronchodilators are:
* Albuterol HFA
* Xopenex HFA
* Berotec
* Brethine Bricanyl, Breathaire
* Proventil HFA
* Ventolin HFA
* Pro-Air HFA
* Maxair

So, where does Combivent come in?

Combivent is both a Preventer and a Rescuer because it contains Atrovent and Albuterol.

Maximum Delivery to the Lungs

If you're feeling the spray of your inhaled medicine on your tongue or in the back of your throat, that means it's not all getting down to your lungs. Using a spacer or a holding chamber can help you get as much inhaled medicine as possible deep into your lungs where it will do the most good.

Check with a respiratory care professional (a licensed Respiratory Therapist or nurse who specializes in COPD), show them your inhaler technique and ask if you can improve upon it. Ask also what special precautions you should take to prevent unwanted side-effects, such as mouth infections or raspy throat.

Timing

If your medicines are in different categories, general consensus is that it's all right to take them one right after the other. Just don't take two medicines that are in the same category at the same time, for example, Albuterol and Proventil, because they both contain Albuterol and that would be overdosing. That said, professional opinions do differ when it comes to timing. Check with your respiratory health professional about when to take each of your inhaled medications for maximum benefit, for your individual situation.

Medicines You Swallow

Because you swallow medications that are in the form of a tablet or capsule, they have to go first through your digestive system. Along the way, they can cause some side effects; more so than the inhaled medicines that go straight to the source of the problem, your lungs. However, oral medications still have their place in helping you breathe.

Prednisone is often used if you have a bad breathing episode. It works very well, within a day or two, and is then tapered down once the exacerbation has passed. Long-term use of oral prednisone should be avoided if at all possible; but if you have severe COPD, are on maximum use of inhalers, and you're still having trouble getting through your day, you may need to be on a low dose daily prednisone.

Methylxanthines

These medicines have been around for a long time and were some of the first effective breathing medications. They work well for some people but are not often prescribed.

Methylxanthines are:
* Theophylline
* Uniphyl

That's about it for the very basics of COPD medications. Remember what we said about fire? Do all you can to prevent one, and hopefully you won't have to do a whole lot of rescuing. It's important for you, a person with COPD, to know – and understand – how your breathing medications work. Once you do, you'll be much closer to controlling your breathing – and your life!

Your Turn

Key points, or … If you don't remember anything else from this chapter, remember this:

- It is your job to understand not only what each breathing medication is supposed to do, but how it is supposed to do it. You're smart enough to understand this!
- Take your preventer medicines as prescribed, every day, even when you're breathing well. They will help keep your breathing stable.
- Have a respiratory care professional observe the technique you use in taking your inhaled

medicines. If you need improvement, he or she will give you suggestions about how to get as much benefit as you can from your inhaled medicines.

Ask yourself this:

- Do I know how my different breathing medications work?
- Am I using the best possible technique?

This week:

- Make sure you're taking your preventer medications exactly as prescribed. If you have questions, ask your doctor or respiratory health professional.

Here's more help

- COPD Medication Guidelines
  http://www.cchs.net/health/health-info/
  docs/2400/2406.asp?index=8698

Hope
[JVT]

It has never been, and never will be, easy work! But the road that is built in hope is more pleasant to the traveler than the road built in despair, even though they both lead to the same destination.
– Marion Zimmer Bradley

Receiving a diagnosis of COPD can be devastating. As patients, we learn that we have a progressive, incurable disease, one that no doubt will alter our life by limiting our physical abilities with shortness of breath and fatigue. We may hear all or none of this information at the point of diagnosis. Some of us are just left to fend for ourselves. Most doctors – even pulmonologists – do not have the time or inclination to educate patients. So we are left with huge holes in knowledge about COPD and how to manage it. But by far, the worst thing left out of diagnosis is hope. We are rarely advised that we have a right to have hope with COPD.

Even if a doctor suspects that his or her patient may have a poor prognosis, that person is still entitled to hope – that should never be taken away. In my case, I was diagnosed with COPD and told I had between two and five years of life left. That was fourteen years ago! Even though I was prescribed supplemental oxygen 24/7 for the rest of my life (which I've faithfully used all these years), I'm still around, still kicking, still working every day, still very much alive – and glad of it!

Everyone deserves hope! But I had to find my own. I've done some of this by my involvement as an advocate for COPDers. Part of my own hope came from my quest for information about this disease. Part of it, I found by writing my book about living with COPD. Part of it I stumbled upon by seeing others who were worse off than I was. And part of it I gained by having faith in my own ability to overcome obstacles, even those caused by chronic illness. I continue to learn about COPD almost every day, and I'm determined not to give in to it.

The big questions about hope usually come a while after the initial diagnosis, after the shock of being told we have a progressive, incurable disease that's not going to go away. Shock tongue-ties us and prevents our brains from allowing us to reach out for vital information. Then, after the initial numbness wears off a bit, we find ourselves in need of an understanding of what we, and our families, are facing.

Physicians are the ones we turn to most often when we are seized by fear of the unknown. I would like to see all pulmonary physicians add a few more basic facts to their ten-minute visit – to add words of hope by making sure that we, as patients, are aware that our life is not over just because we have COPD. We need to be encouraged to become active in the management of our disease – partners with our doctors – knowing that the goal is now stability of our disease and living as healthy and happy – and hopeful – as possible.

There are many things we can do to keep from getting worse, to prevent us from spiraling downward. We have a lung disease that is chronic and usually progressive but we can choose to live our lives in ways that help us remain stable. By following our doctor's treatment program: eating a healthy diet, keeping up with an exercise routine, getting enough sleep, maintaining a social life, avoiding exposure to viruses and other harmful bugs, and keeping a positive outlook, we are on our way to stability!

When we're beginning to feel helpless we must fight our way back to better control of our lives. How? By finding different ways to accomplish our goals even if we are limited in our physical strength. We may not be able to do what we once did in the same way we did it, but that doesn't mean we can't do lots of things.

No one should be without hope, ever! It's a ladder to hold on to. It is a reason to get up in the mornings. It gives us reason to smile. It lets us reach out to help others. It helps us sleep at night. Having hope gives us insight into what is most important in our lives. But most of all, hope provides us with inspiration, encouragement, and strength to face each day.

Bonus Box
Thoughts on Hope
Steve Rietveld

Growing up just outside Chicago, Steve's life was going along just as planned. He had graduated from high school, had a lot of friends, was involved in activities at church, and had just gone to baseball try-out camp. As an only son, he was poised to carry on the successful family business. But in a moment, his life changed. He was injured while working with his father on the family farm; and the result of his injury was that, at age 20, Steve became a quadriplegic. Although Steve doesn't have pulmonary disease per se, he has experienced numerous health problems over the years, including needing a pacemaker,

---

colostomy, and tracheotomy with oxygen, as well as experiencing several bouts of pneumoniaand a collapsed lung. Nebulizer treatments and suctioning are a routine part of his day. Here are Steve's thoughts on Hope.

As a person with a chronic lung disease, you might think that my injury, leaving me paralyzed, is a very bad thing and worse than what you have, but you cannot look at it that way. Sure, this is a devastating injury, but the main thing is that I still have my mind and *I'm still me*. My body is not disfigured – it still looks the same. It just cannot move. Of course it could be worse: I could be on a respirator, not able to move my arms like I can now, or my mind could be damaged, but none of those things have happened, so I'm very fortunate.

I have discovered the world of computers; they are a godsend – and my link to the outside world. Had I not been injured would I have been this involved with computers? Probably not. If I can inspire or help just one person, with words, comfort, or visiting my website, that's good. Anything I have to share or help people with, I'm happy to give. So, out of a tragedy there have been positives. Don't look at me as a person who has lost so much – but someone who has gained so much more.

And now regarding the subject of Hope. Hope is something that's hard to keep hold of, to keep in your sights when something happens to you – chronic or terminal disease, an accident – anything. At first when something devastating happens you think there is no hope and never will be. Honestly, I did not even want to hope for anything when I waswas first injured. My first thoughts were to pretty much give up because, what was the point? My life was over. My plans were over. My dreams were gone. What good would, or could I be ever again?

With an injury like mine, or a chronic/terminal illness, acceptance of the situation is a key before you can begin to hope. Sure, I hope there will be a cure for paralysis – and I'm sure someday there will be – but not in my lifetime. That doesn't mean I can't hope for something. When news comes out about new research or new discoveries, it's easy to think it will be available the next day. In truth, it could still be years away and so I have to hope – in perspective. I'm thankful for even small advances that help me deal with day-to-day living, even if it is not a cure. I can even be hopeful for something as simple as having a good day.

We've always got to have hope…have to keep that flame burning. A lot of days this is easier said than done. The sun will keep on rising every day and we never know what that day will bring. But we have to hope that it will be good. This is why I will never give up or lose hope, because I want to be around to experience everything I can.

Whether you are spiritual or not, hope can still be there. On the coldest, darkest days of winter we still hope for spring. Finally, it comes. You know how you feel when you see that first flower pushing up through the snow? Without hope we have nothing. If life is a game of cards I have been dealt this hand. It's not the hand I wanted, but I will play it, I will make the best of it, and I'll never lose hope.

Your Turn

Key points, or...If you don't remember anything else from this chapter, remember this:

- Along with receiving a COPD diagnosis, you and your doctor should talk about what you can hope for.
- It is good, and it is right, to have hope – for something – no matter how small, no matter how bad things are.

Ask yourself this:

- What can I hope for? Is there something coming up that I can look forward to?

This week:

- Wake up with one new hope, no matter how small, for that day.

Here's more help

- *A Grace Disguised: How the Soul Grows Through Loss* (includes Steve's story and others), by Jerry Sittser
- *The Anatomy of Hope,* by Jerome Groopman, MD.
- *Finding Hope: Ways to See Life in a Brighter Light,* by James E Miller and Ronna Jevne
- *Hope For The Flowers,* by Trina Paulus

Worry
[Vijai Sharma, Ph.D.]

Worry is interest paid on trouble before it comes due.
– William Ralph Inge

The origin of the word "worry" offers interesting insights regarding the nature and function of worry. The English words, "worrowen," "wirien," "Wyrgan," mean "to choke" or "to strangle." In Medieval English the verb "worry" also meant "to gnaw," or to continually bite or tear something. Worries and chronic anxiety gnaw at us and, bit by bit, wear away our inner security and peace of mind.

You may be a person with COPD who had an anxiety disorder prior to developing COPD, or developed one after the onset of the lung impairment. You may have had a Generalized Anxiety Disorder (GAD) from very early on, long before you developed COPD.

You may have been born with what is called anxious temperament. According to temperament related research, perhaps 20% of children are born with anxious temperament. Out of the 20% anxious temperament children, some will develop one or more anxiety spectrum disorders, notably GAD, phobias, panic attacks, or Obsessive-Compulsive Disorder. If you have excessive anxiety or concern associated with breathing difficulty, you should get an evaluation for a possible underlying disorder.

In some cases, worrying is a symptom of an anxiety disorder, depressive disorder, or a result of a deeply painful life event, such as betrayal of trust, abandonment, severe humiliation, or abuse.

If you're a worrier, you should know that to a great extent, you have a choice regarding what you think. You have the power to fight off negative and disturbing thoughts that invade your mind. You can do this by learning what you're dealing with, facing the worry monster, and breaking the hold it has on you.

Worrying is to chew over and over again that which has already been chewed. Worrying has a repetitive and obsessive quality about it. A worrier is fixated on negative outcomes and possible pitfalls. A worrier imagines every misfortune that might come along. Oh, those errors, accidents, and all possible bad things that can go wrong! Remember, some of our demons are of our own making.

Do you have a worry problem?

* Have you begun to worry more than you ever did?
* Do you worry more than others do?
* Do you tend to multiply the possibilities of what can go wrong?
* On an average day over the past month, what percentage of the day did you feel worried?
* Have you frequently been so worried that you kept tossing and turning in bed and couldn't sleep?
* Have you ever been told, "Stop worrying! Relax!"

If you answered "yes" to any of these questions, *don't worry*, we will provide tips to help you cut down on your worry time. Read on!

I am sure that after worrying all night long you find yourself in the morning exactly in the same situation you were in the night before, except more sleepy and tired! In spite of worrying all night, you didn't solve anything, learn anything new, or acquire any possession, except perhaps a headache. God gave us the ability to worry to help us assess the risks facing us, and to plan appropriate steps to meet our needs. The purpose of the "work of worrying" is summarized in the saying, "forewarned is forearmed!" But if you worry only, and don't take the required action, you never get out of the swirling waters onto the shore.

The One-Minute Manager – Tips for cutting down on the habit of worrying

If you are a chronic worrier, it means that through the practice of many years of worrying, you have become really good at it. The mind learns to have "worry spasms," or a kind of "brain hiccups" that just refuse to quit. The first few seconds you start worrying are critical to stop the ever-growing worry web. When the first worry thought strikes you, you have just a few seconds, a maximum of one minute, to break the chain of worry thoughts before your entire mind is involved in it. Once you are too involved with your worrying thoughts, you end up in the "worry grip!" Once you're there, you might not be able to relax for the next several hours – or even the whole night.

It helps to think of worry as if it's a small patch of weeds in the spring. Before you know it weeds can take over the whole garden; but you can get rid of them if you apply weed killer as soon as you see them sprout. You can break a single stick with ease; it's difficult to break a bunch of them together.

When your mind becomes involved with the action of worrying, the body gets involved, as well. You tense up and the level of stress hormones keep rising, which fuels worrying thoughts non-stop. You can train yourself to stop worrying. Just as you train your muscles to learn a golf swing, train your brain to take a swing at the worry monster.

Here are some tips to stop the worry thoughts:

1. As soon as you catch the first worry thought, challenge it! Say something positive to yourself right away. Offer counter evidence to oppose the main thrust of your worry thoughts. Offer yourself thoughts that negate your worst fears.

2. Imagine all possible outcomes instead of the negative ones. Challenge "What if…?" thoughts with "So what…" thoughts. Also challenge your negative thinking with a skeptical attitude and ask "How so?"

   Here is an example:

   Worry thought: What if they don't come to see me anymore?

   Counter thought: So what if they don't come to see me anymore. I can do without them.

   Worry thought: They may all be tired of me.

   Counter thought: How so? I feel they genuinely care about me.

   Turn the tables on your worry thoughts!

3. If you've tried everything else and you still can't shake off your worry thoughts, get out of bed and write them down. After you write them down, read them to yourself. You may often find that your imagination is somewhat exaggerated.

4. When a worry strikes you, do something physical for five minutes, such as stretch, hum, or whistle. Then sit down and write about what worried you and the actions you can take to address that problem. Note the earliest time when you can act on them.
5. Think of a positive self-affirming thought. For example, "I am a doer, not a worrier!"
6. Blow your breath into your palms and say to yourself, "I just blew off my worry," and go to bed. The next morning, follow the actions you wrote down.

If you don't strike quickly at them, worries multiply, adding to an ever-growing list of things to worry about. We worry about everything, ranging from things less likely to happen to those that are most unlikely to happen. All things are not lions and tigers, but they may *appear* so to us. Soon, the world seems to be a dangerous place. Previously, one sensed danger from just a few sources; now he or she sees it everywhere. There is no shortcut and no easy way out. The dragons need to be slain one by one.

Chronic and excessive worrying can isolate you from others, stripping you of your social support system. Don't get so involved in the act of worrying that you can't find time to connect with others. Don't let worry isolate you from people who love you!

You can learn to extricate your life from the clutches of anxiety. You probably underestimate your own power and overestimate the danger of things that confront you. If you need to, see a therapist. If there is a traumatic event in your past that keeps gnawing at you, work through it with a counselor. Often the way to overcome pain is through it and not around it.

Give yourself a gift: Learn ways to calm your fears. As you involve yourself in new situations and new activities, preoccupation with anxiety will decrease. As you develop greater self-confidence and find your life more satisfying, you may not even need anxiety medication.

Knowing you have the power to choose your thoughts is one of the best kept secrets! You do have a choice regarding what you think and how you feel. Just because you have always thought and felt a certain way, doesn't mean you can't train yourself to think differently. You may not have power over the outside world, but you have the choice to decide what thoughts you think – and the power to beat the worry monster.

Your Turn

Key points, or . . . If you don't remember anything else from this chapter, remember this:

- If you are a chronic worrier, with or without COPD, you can learn to control your worry.
- You can choose your thoughts.
- Worry can affect your physical as well as emotional health and well-being.
- It is important to stop the worry quickly after it starts.

Ask yourself this:

- Do I have a worry problem?

This week:

- Write down your three major worries.

- Write down your "worry thoughts" related to each of the three major worries.
- Write down your "counter thoughts" for three major "worry thoughts."

Here's more help

- *Quiet Your Mind: An Easy-to-Use Guide to Ending Chronic Worry and Negative Thoughts and Living a Calmer Life,* by John Selby
- *The Worry Workbook: Twelve Steps to Anxiety-Free Living,* by Les Carter, PH.D and Frank Minirth, MD

Excerpted from *Overcoming Anxiety and Depression – Breathing Correctly in COPD/ Emphysema: A Self Care Book for People with COPD and a Psychosocial Manual for Professionals,* intended for future publication. Copyright©2008, Vijai Sharma,PhD. (all inquiries to be directed to dr.sharma@mindpub.com)

End-Stage COPD: What is it and What Does it Mean for Me?

[JMM]

In the face of uncertainty,
there is nothing wrong with hope.
– Bernie S. Siegel, MD

"You have end-stage COPD," is possibly one of the most frightening – and confusing – words a person can hear.

This week we're going to talk about three simple steps that anyone who has heard these dreaded words – and anyone with chronic lung disease for that matter – should follow.

1. Get the Facts Straight

When someone, anyone, tells you you're at a certain stage of a disease, ask questions. Find out what it is that determines that stage; and next, where you fit in.

The very first question I ask when a new patient comes in to pulmonary rehab is, "What has the doctor told you about what's going on in your lungs?" How the patient answers this question tells me a lot about what he or she has been told about their lung disease, what they understand about it, and what it means to them. Most of the time when I ask this, I find that the patient doesn't know a whole lot. So, we sit down and take a look at the pulmonary function test results and see what's what.

2. Know and Understand Your Numbers

If your doctor gives you a number from the result of your pulmonary function test, or spirometry, he or she will probably tell you a percentage. For instance, "You have 50% of your lung function left." Some people think that if they have been told they have 50% lung function, it means they have one good lung and one bad lung. Not so.

Here's what we're talking about when it comes to percentage: Before you perform the lung function test, the technician enters information into the computer – your age, height, gender, and race. The pulmonary function machine knows what flow rates, volumes, and functions a person with those same characteristics with healthy lungs, would achieve. These lung function values are called *normal predicted*.

You do the test – all that breathing in and blowing out – and your results are then compared to the ideal (*normal predicted*) lung function numbers. For example, if a person your age, height, gender and race with good lungs would blow out two liters and you, with your best effort, exhale one liter, your number on that maneuver would be half of *normal predicted*, or 50%. Most likely, both your lungs are diseased and have a limited ability to perform.

Now let's look at the stages of COPD related to those numbers. If you have COPD, one very important function of your lungs is the FEV_1. This is the Forced Expiratory Volume in one second. This is the amount of air you blow out in the very first second of your long exhalation.

Classification of COPD by Severity[5]

Stage 0: At Risk
Chronic cough and sputum production; lung function is still normal.

---

5. GOLD (Global Initiative for Chronic Obstructive Lung Disease) Guidelines, evidence-based guidelines for COPD diagnosis, management, and prevention. http://www.goldcopd.com

Stage I: Mild COPD
FEV_1 – at least 80% of normal predicted. You may or may not notice symptoms.
Stage II: Moderate COPD
FEV_1 – between 50% and 80% of normal predicted. You usually have some shortness of breath with exertion; and may or may not have a chronic cough.
Stage III: Severe COPD
FEV_1 – between 30% and 50% of normal predicted. You are often tired and short of breath and may have frequent exacerbations – episodes of worse breathing – requiring extra treatment or even hospitalization.
Stage IV: Very Severe (sometimes called end-stage) COPD
FEV_1 – less than 30% of normal predicted. You may often be short of breath, even at rest.

It's important to know that one person's numbers don't mean the same thing for another. We're all different. I've known people with 30% lung function who struggle to walk twenty feet, and those who have 19% lung function who move about relatively well. So, although it's important to know your lung function numbers and understand what they mean, you must also realize that your lung function numbers not only do not define what you can or cannot do, but most of all, how long you're going to live.

3. Don't Give Up!

Before you phone your local monument company to have them carve tomorrow's date on your gravestone, know that with proper care and treatment you can live for many years with very limited lung function! The term "end-stage" is just a term, based on the perspective of who you're talking to. For example, a respiratory therapist who works day after day with severe, but stable, COPD patients in pulmonary rehabilitation probably has a much different take on your prognosis than a doctor or nurse who sees pulmonary patients only when they are sick.

In doing research for this piece, I read an article written by a home care nurse who talked about patients with less than 30% lung function as being end-stage and barely able to walk more than a couple of steps. Again, I can tell you that there are many patients in pulmonary rehab with less than 25% lung function who do very well! So, no, being told you have end-stage COPD is not a death sentence. There is a lot you can do, and you can live a long time. Next week we'll talk specifically about how you can do all right, in spite of being labeled as "end-stage."

Your Turn

Key points, or . . . If you don't remember anything else from this chapter, remember this:

- Being told that you have end-stage COPD is not a death sentence!
- Two people with the same pulmonary function numbers are not necessarily in the same physical condition. Their breathing can differ significantly.
- You can live a long time with advanced COPD, if you learn how to best manage it.

Ask yourself this:

- Do you know your current FEV_1 number, and what it was a year ago?

This week:

- If you have COPD and have not had a pulmonary function complete test or spirometry within the last year, call your doctor and ask him or her to order one.

Here's more help

- *Huffin' n' Puffin': Living with COPD,* by Leland Gordon Vogel
- Olivia's Pages, "End Stage"http://www.olivija.com/endstage/

End-Stage COPD: Staying Healthy
[JMM]

Your future depends on many things, but mostly on you.
– Frank Tyger

Last week we talked about end-stage COPD, what it is and what it means for you. We learned that in spite of what it sounds like, end-stage is *not a death sentence*! On the contrary, you can live for many years, and do pretty well, with this diagnosis. You may be thinking, "So, if end-stage doesn't mean the end of my world, then what *does* it mean? How can I make the most of my life now – and for the rest of my life?"

Before we talk about that, here's one very important thing to remember: As far as your day-to-day life goes, in some ways your life with severe COPD will probably never be the same, as the life you once had. It might be a different life, but that doesn't mean it can't be a good life. There are many things you can do to make your life healthy, joyful, and even fun, when you have end-stage COPD.

Stay Healthy

COPD is a disease, but not necessarily an illness. Yes, you have this disease, but that doesn't mean you have to be sick. The most important thing you can do when you have severe COPD is to avoid what we call an "acute exacerbation" of COPD – a bad episode of worse breathing and potentially serious illness.

You can do this by:

1. Knowing your triggers – things that make your breathing suddenly worse
2. Recognizing early warning signs – signals that you might be headed for an acute exacerbation. (See chapters: January – Week 4 and September – Week 3) If you know what to watch for, you have a much better chance of staying healthy, avoiding pneumonia, staying out of the hospital, and just getting on with life.

Quit Smoking

If you were a smoker and you've already quit, good for you! If you haven't, you may be thinking, "What the heck, it's too late anyway." Please know this – it's never too late to quit! In fact, smoking cessation is looked upon by COPD experts as the number one "disease altering therapy." And who wouldn't want to alter the course of a progressive disease? If you're struggling with weight loss, smoking cessation will help you keep those much-needed pounds on board. If you quit, your cough will mostly likely decrease and you'll be better able to fight infections. And if you slip back and start smoking again, just make a new plan, get back up on that horse and try again. Don't give up! You can do it!

Be Informed

Don't be at the mercy of the mystery of lung disease! Take control of your life by learning what's going on in your lungs. Learn correct breathing techniques. Make sure you know exactly how your inhalers work, which ones are maintenance and which ones are rescuers, (see chapter July – Week 5) and how to get as much benefit from them as possible. Be skeptical of treatments or remedies that claim to cure your disease. If it sounds too good to be true, it probably is (see chapter September – Week 2)! People with COPD who seek information and learn from it do far better than those who don't.

Connect with Others

Isolating yourself and being anxious and depressed can make you feel even worse. There's more to life than sitting in your chair and watching TV. Below are three ways to connect with others for education and support. Choose at least one – you'll be so glad you did!

Get into Pulmonary Rehab

As much as you might be tempted to shuffle over to your recliner, plop down and stay there for good, don't do it! Pulmonary Rehabilitation is a program of exercise and education especially designed for people with COPD (see chapter January – Week 5). In pulmonary rehab you'll gain strength, stamina, and flexibility, learn about your lungs and how to stay as healthy as possible. You'll discover the right way to breathe, how to pace yourself, conserve energy, eat right, and relax. You will learn about exercise and activity – what is safe and what is not – and what you should or shouldn't do to stay as healthy as possible.

To start, you need a doctor's order and a lung function test done within the last year. If the doctor or respiratory staff at your local hospital doesn't know where the nearest pulmonary rehab program is located, check with the American Association of Cardiovascular and Pulmonary Rehabilitation (AACVPR). Contact information is at the end of this chapter.

Join a Better Breathers' Club

At a Better Breathers' support group you will learn from guest speakers about staying healthy with COPD and meet people with similar concerns. Your spouse or support person might also connect with someone who understands the unique issues of a caregiver / well spouse. Attending a breathing support group is free of charge and does not require a doctor's order. For the breathing support group nearest you call your local hospital, oxygen supply company, or visit the American Lung Association (ALA) website. Information is at the end of this chapter.

Join an Online COPD Community

You can find lots of information and support online. Pulmonary websites and Internet communities contain not only loads of solid information about living well with COPD, but you'll also meet folks just like you who are living every day with COPD. Forums are open twenty-four hours a day to ask questions, get encouragement and support, and even share a laugh! Don't go it alone! Becoming part of a group – Pulmonary Rehabilitation, Better Breathers' or one online – will lighten your load, help you feel better, and breathe easier.

Your Turn

Key points, or . . . If you don't remember anything else from this chapter, remember this:

- If you have end-stage COPD, you don't have to stay at home and be sick much of the time.
- There is a lot you can do to stay healthy and be in control of your life.
- There are many people out there who have the same concerns that you have.

Ask yourself this:

- Am I connected with a pulmonary rehab program, local breathing support group, or online COPD community?

This week:

- If you're not connected with one of the above, make it happen. If you already are, read one article or chapter in a COPD book, magazine, or online, about living well with COPD.

Here's more help

- To find a Pulmonary Rehabilitation Program near you, visit http://www.aacvpr.org. Phone: 312-321-5146 / Email: aacvpr@aacvpr.org
- To find a Better Breather's Club near you, go to the American Lung Association website, http://www.lungusa.org , or check your phone book for your state or local American Lung Association office. To call: 1-800-LUNGUSA (586-4872).
- An online community can be found on Breathing Better Living Well, http://www.breathingbetterlivingwell.com.
- For more help, read or review the chapters mentioned in the text of this chapter.

End-Stage COPD:
Happy at Home and Away
[JMM]

*There are many wonderful things that will
never be done if you do not do them.*
– Charles D. Gil

When you have severe, or end-stage COPD (I hate that term!) yes, it's important to do your best to stay healthy, physically, but we should never underestimate the value of emotional health. Below is some wisdom on how to live a full and happy life from those who know – people with end-stage COPD. All these suggestions might not work for you, but if you try just one or two, you might be surprised how much better you'll feel.

Get out there!

It might take some effort, but make plans to go out regularly; to dinner, to your grandchild's sports event or school program, or even for a ride in the car. Feeling self-conscious about wearing your oxygen? Would you expect someone who needs glasses to drive without them? Of course not! If your doctor says you need supplemental oxygen, wear it. You'll breathe easier and put a lot less stress on your heart, your brain and the rest of your body. If someone has a problem with you wearing oxygen, it's their problem – not yours.

Don't sweat the small stuff

It may be a cliché, but really…when something starts to bug you, ask yourself, "Does it really matter all that much? Is this that much of a biggie, or can I just let it go?" Being anxious can lead to even worse shortness of breath. The simple serenity prayer offers great advice: *God grant me the serenity to accept the things I cannot change; courage to change the things I can; and wisdom to know the difference.*

Laugh

Make smiles and laughter – and sharing them – a priority. One of my most favorite things about working with people with COPD is the fun we have together, telling jokes, laughing and kidding around. Truly, some of the best times I've ever had are when I'm in a room full of people with end-stage COPD.

Record your history

Everyone has a story to tell, and we should all pass ours along, whatever our age – or our health status. Make plans with a friend or family member (maybe a grandchild), to listen as you tell your story while they record it on audio, video, or digitally. Just sit down and start talking. You'll be so glad you did!

Help others

When I was writing my first book I asked pulmonary patients this question: "If you could say one thing to someone with chronic lung disease who is about to give up, what would you say?" One lady with very severe lung disease said, "Do something to help someone." Wow.

Make a phone call or send a cheerful note to someone who's feeling down. Volunteer for your local hospital or public library by doing a sit-down job. Read to a child. Give someone a ride to the grocery store or the doctor's office. Even if you're short of breath you can help yourself – by helping others.

Go with the flow

Probably one of the biggest concerns of COPD patients – and the most confusing – is the mystery of good days and bad days. Yes, it's important to pay attention to changes in your breathing, but don't spend too much emotional energy trying to figure out why yesterday was so good and today is not. Many times there is simply no explanation. Just accept that bad days are a fact of life and know that tomorrow will probably be better.

One way to make the most of bad breathing days is to have a box or basket stocked with quiet activities you don't always have time for – a book or magazine to read, word puzzles, jigsaw puzzles, a movie you've been meaning to watch, or a small sewing or sit-down repair project. (See chapter February – Week 3.)

Go on vacation

Are you kidding? No, I'm not. Sure, traveling with any chronic disease takes planning, but if at all possible, take that trip! You'll be getting out, seeing something new, having fun, and making memories to keep.

For many people with end-stage COPD, moving around is a big effort. In a swimming pool you'll have the freedom to move around smoothly and easily. And yes, you can swim while wearing oxygen! If you have trouble walking a distance, rent a wheel chair or a scooter. The goal is to enjoy a getaway and see some sites – not to struggle with your breathing. Check these resources for more travel tips and ideas.

* Travel Tips from the Cleveland Clinic http://my.clevelandclinic.org/disorders/Chronic -- Obstructive -- Pulmonary -- Disease -- copd/ hic -- Traveling -- Tips -- for -- People -- with -- COPD.aspx
Travel tips from COPD International
* http://www.copd-international.com/Library/ traveling.htm
Sea Puffers Cruises for people with pulmonary disease offers you the support you need to travel with oxygen. 866-673-3019.
http://www.seapuffers.com/

Don't Give Up – and Don't Forget to Live!

When you have very severe or end-stage COPD – whatever you call it – sure, there are things you can no longer do the way you once did, *but there are still many things you can accomplish and enjoy.* Whatever you do, don't forget to live! You can live long – and well – with end-stage COPD.

New Perspectives
[JVT]

Compassion for everyone is the basic principle
that leads to peace and happiness.
– Buddha

Do you ever take the time to reflect on how living with a chronic disease has affected you? I don't mean the loss of things we can no longer do because of our physical restrictions. We all put in our grieving time for those losses, and most of us do our best to open new doors and find new activities we can involve ourselves in, even with our disease. (I now count three chronic diseases in my own life – COPD, diabetes, and Post Polio Syndrome).

What I'm writing about today is that the way we look at others may have changed. Can you see a change in your feelings toward others, or a major shift in priorities since you were diagnosed?

It's funny how when we are faced with illness and / or disability life has a way of teaching us some very good lessons, whether we want them or not. We learn the value of life, and how we should never take it for granted. We learn that life is fragile, and that we – all of us – are mortal. We learn about patience and lifestyle adjustments, and about the importance of taking an active role in the management of our wellness.

I think though, for me, one of the most lasting things I have learned from being someone with chronic disease is compassion. In the ten years since I've been diagnosed with COPD, my personality has changed. I am now less judgmental. I can empathize with those faced with a serious illness or disease. My heart goes out to a person with a disability of any kind. I'm more willing to lend a helping hand or a sympathetic ear to others who are ill, especially those with lung disease. I like to think of it as a patient developing more patience. And I believe this all translates into compassion.

I've learned, too, that through the involvement with my support group I have found great joy in helping other COPD patients. And I know that in helping others, it gives me back so much more than I give – even the power to heal – if not my body, my spirit.

What about you? Has having COPD caused you to become more sensitive in dealing with others? Has it helped you to be more gentle and caring? Has it made you better understand someone else's challenges? Has it made you more grateful, more patient, and more compassionate?

Being mindful of other people's feelings and needs helps us become less centered on our problems – and it certainly makes us easier to be around! It opens doors to new understanding, and helps bring peace to our own state of mind. Just think of the good you can do by opening those doors; the help you can bring, the comfort you can give to others. And when we help others we help ourselves as well.

Your Turn

Key points, or … If you don't remember anything else from this chapter, remember this:

- Having COPD, or other chronic disease, can cause you to become more understanding, patient, caring and compassionate.

Ask yourself this:

- How have I changed, as a person, since being diagnosed with COPD?

This week:

- Do something kind for a person who is in need of understanding or help. Write down what you did and how it made you feel.

Here's more help

- *The Complete Guide to Understanding and Living with COPD: From A COPDer's Perspective,* by R.D. Martin
- From COPD Health Center on MSN: "My COPD Story: From Patient to Patience" by Jeff Shumaker http://health-tools.health.msn.com/copd/from-patient-to-patience

Have I Got a Cure for You! Understanding Alternative Treatments for COPD

[Dr. Robert Sandhaus, MD, PhD, FCCP]

Only a fool tests the depth of the water with both feet.
— African Proverb

As a respiratory therapist I'm often asked about alternative treatments for COPD such as herbs, vitamins, mechanical breathing aides, breathing techniques, body manipulation, massage, etc. Sometimes the advertising – and the testimonials – sound so convincing. What should patients believe? To sort it all out, I consulted pulmonary expert, Dr. Robert "Sandy" Sandhaus, MD, PhD, FCCP, of National Jewish Health, the number one respiratory hospital in the United States. Think of these expert answers the next time you're wondering if an alternative treatment is right for you.

1. Whenever I hear about something other than a "traditional" medicine for COPD, my doctor tells me it's no good. C'mon, aren't the big drug companies just saying these new methods are no good simply to keep us buying their products?

I think everyone wants to find ways to help or cure disease that are mild, "natural," and non-injurious. Because of this, there is a tendency to head toward alternative treatments, especially if more traditional therapies are either not working well for you, or are causing side effects that seem worse than the disease. The challenge is to know what works and what doesn't – for you – and making choices from among the hundreds of agents and claims of success.

The reason most doctors are much more comfortable with "traditional" medications and therapies is that they have been tested, evaluated, approved, and often retested over and over, to find the best doses and combinations. The initial source of these medications may well be an herb or other agent that might have been considered "alternative" in the past.

Other medications are based on a scientific understanding of disease mechanisms and actions. These two methods of discovering new drugs are well represented in COPD therapies. Still, COPD deaths have been rising and there are many individuals who still have severe symptoms, in spite of regular use of traditional medications.

Given the above, it would be great to have a natural or herbal remedy that one could take which would make their COPD significantly improve. One may exist somewhere. The question is how would we know? Alternative medications don't have to undergo the traditional testing and retesting, study and re-study, that traditional medicines do.

In general, the success stories are either by word of mouth or by an "expert" trying to sell a product or program, often with dramatic claims of success. It seems unlikely that all the claims and stories are true; otherwise there would be a lot of cured COPD patients out there. So how do you choose? I just don't have an answer to that question.

In addition, there is a growing appreciation that some herbal or alternative medications can actually lead to quite significant side effects and especially, dangerous interactions with other medications, whether traditional or alternative.

Finally, there is the question of whether docs and drug companies actually know how to cure COPD but won't do it, because they want their patients to keep coming back to provide income or the drug companies just want to sell their medications. Certainly, drug companies do want to make money! But, speaking as a doctor who treats patients with COPD every day, if I could prescribe or recommend a medication that cured COPD, I would be the happiest doctor in the world.

2. What's wrong with using herbal remedies for pulmonary problems? Herbs are natural so they can't hurt me, isn't that right?

Herbs may be just fine. Nevertheless, the fact that something is an herb doesn't guarantee it is either safe or effective. As mentioned above, herbs can interact with other medications both natural and traditional. Don't forget that most poisons were also initially isolated from plants and herbs.

3. What about some breathing methods offered in seminars? They come from countries other than the United States. Are we in the United States just being self-centered, believing that only we have all the answers?

Breathing exercise and training have an important place in many pulmonary diseases, especially COPD. Many pulmonary rehabilitation programs incorporate a variety of methods into their instruction. Several studies have evaluated non-traditional breathing methods, such as Yoga and Buteyko, as an adjunct to COPD therapy. The studies have shown mixed results.

In part, this appears to be due to the fact that some methods, like Buteyko, have no standardized methodology and often include components that are educational and nutritional. While studies have shown less bronchodilator usage in patients instructed in some form of Buteyko, there has been no change in their lung function or exercise tolerance. Often the control group also has a strong positive response, although not as dramatic as the treatment group, suggesting that just getting into a program that takes an interest in your overall health is beneficial to a COPD patient.

4. I've seen some books that talk about COPD being curable. In just one quick search I found several articles that came up when I entered "COPD Cure."

What can I say? I hope the whole world is cured of its COPD by one of these programs. I know that many claim they have done scientific studies to prove their effectiveness – things like sheep stem cells injected into the lungs in a clinic in Mexico, and oxidant or anti-oxidant medications that allow the lung to repair its damage. Not only do these therapies and studies not stand up to close evaluation, they may well be quite harmful to those taking them. Finally, when you actually contact the centers offering these cures, you find that many want a substantial, up-front cash payment. This should make you very suspicious.

5. What about Vitamin "O" or oxygen drops to improve your oxygen levels? I got something in the mail with

testimonials about how this helps people breathe better and I know someone personally who says he thinks it helps.

One of the biggest scams in the alternative medication arena centers on the promotion of oxygen preparations taken by mouth. Whether drinks, drops, pills or capsules, there is no true scientific evidence of benefit and the rationale behind them is highly suspect – some may even do harm (in addition to the damage to your wallet).

First, there is no evidence that there is any significant uptake of oxygen in the stomach or intestines, even if you could deliver oxygen there. The air sacs in the lungs are microscopically thin so oxygen can cross their specialized membrane to move from the lungs into the blood. The stomach and intestines have no such apparatus to allow for the easy passage of oxygen.

Second, the ways that these products deliver "oxygen" is highly suspect. Among the products claiming to provide increased oxygen, the delivery approaches include making the solution high in dissolved oxygen, the addition of "oxygen generating" chemicals, and the addition of minerals that have oxygen in their formula. The most common mineral on earth, silicon dioxide (sand), has two oxygen molecules in its formula, but that doesn't mean it will deliver oxygen to your body – so don't eat it!

You can make a solution that has extra oxygen dissolved in it by bubbling oxygen through it, especially at high pressure. But after you've done that if you leave the solution exposed to air, it will lose all the extra oxygen in a matter of minutes. The most common chemical used as an oxygen generate is hydrogen peroxide, a chemical well known as a potent oxidant. Sure, it generates oxygen, but a very caustic, free-radical type.

The claims advertised for these oxygen liquids include, in addition to increasing the oxygen in your blood, the ability to kill cancer cells, bacterial viruses, and toxins. Most websites advertising these products make claims that bacteria, germs, and cancer cells can't survive when there is plenty of oxygen around. Actually, most cancer cells and bacteria LOVE oxygen and will grow more vigorously in its presence.

So why are there people who swear by these products? Probably because there are a certain number of people who will feel better with any new therapy. There is the "placebo effect" as one explanation. Another is that some people feel better when they take responsibility for their own care. Finally, there are some who would have started feeling better anyway, and the taking of this medication coincided with their feeling better.

This is one class of alternative therapies I'd recommend avoiding.

6. What about Omega-3 Fatty Acids? I've been hearing more about that helping people with pulmonary disease. Mary Pierce (patient with Alpha-1 and recipient of a highly successful double-lung transplant) talked about it years ago and now I'm hearing that they really are helpful in pulmonary disease – or is this more related to prevention?

Omega-3 Fatty Acids are a necessary dietary component and there is growing evidence of its anti-inflammatory and other beneficial effects. Its actual role in lung disease is unclear at this time but, since COPD and many other lung diseases have inflammation as a prominent component, this may well prove an effective adjunctive therapy. Besides, I'd never disagree with Mary Pierce!

Dr. Robert Sandhaus is Professor of Medicine and the Director of the Alpha-1 Antitrypsin Deficiency Program at the National Jewish Medical and Research Center in Denver, Colorado. He is the Clinical Director of the Alpha-1 Foundation and the Medical Director and Executive Vice President of AlphaNet based in Miami, Florida.

Your Turn

Key points, or … If you don't remember anything else from this chapter, remember this:

- You should not believe everything you read or hear about new treatments for COPD.
- Untraditional therapies are often put into practice before they are widely tested.
- Unscrupulous people tend to target those who are desperate for relief from symptoms.

Ask yourself this:

- Have the medications and therapies I take for my COPD been proven safe and effective?

This week:

- If you currently take, or are considering trying an alternative therapy, ask your doctor if it is safe and effective.

Here's more help

- Quackwatch. http://www.quackwatch.com
- "COPD Alternative Treatments" http://www.healthline.com/health/copd-alternative-treatments

- *Your Guide to Alternative Medicine: Understanding, Locating, and Selecting Holistic Treatment and Practitioners,* by Larry P. Credit and Margaret J. Nowak

Facing Fall

Preventing Exacerbations and when to Call the Doctor

[JMM]

To our friends in the Southern Hemisphere: This week, read May – Week 3: Gardening and Yard Work

An ounce of prevention is worth a pound of cure.
– Benjamin Franklin

"Stat – neb treatment and ABGs in the emergency room – stat – neb treatment and ABGs in the emergency room." The voice of the ER unit secretary came across my pager.

It was 10:00pm on a cool autumn night, at the start of flu season. I walked into ER Room Six to find Steve, a man in his mid sixties, sitting on the edge of the gurney, leaning forward, coughing hard and struggling to breathe. I took a sample of arterial blood to test his oxygen and carbon dioxide levels, and put it on ice. I'd run the sample later, but right now the most important thing was to give Steve some relief. I handed him a hand-held nebulizer, already misting with a medicine to open his lungs. He put it to his mouth and breathed it in.

I patted his shoulder and said, "Not doing too well tonight, are you? Have you been sick for a while?"

"Nope. I was…fine until…tonight. This came…out of…nowhere."

"Hmmmm…" I said. "Have you been coughing any more than usual over the last few days?"

Taking deeper breaths now and looking a bit more comfortable, Steve nodded.

"Have you been coughing anything up?"

"Well, yeah…"

"Was it any different than usual? Did it have color to it? Was it thick and sticky?" I asked.

Steve gave me kind of a dirty look, like I'd asked a weird question; to those outside the respiratory world, it probably was. Then he said, "Come to think of it… I've been coughing up green stuff…for about a week."

Steve was not a stupid man, nor was he careless. He had recently quit smoking and generally took pretty good care of himself, but he had no idea – no one ever told him – that especially for him, a person with COPD, a change in cough and a change in the color of mucus is just one major, early warning sign of lung infection. If Steve had known not only what to watch for, but sought help at the first sign of trouble, he'd probably be at home right now resting, able to make it through this infection with a day or two off work, instead of in the ER. Now, he was facing a three-day hospital stay and a week off of work.

One of the biggest concerns for a person with COPD is becoming sick, having an acute exacerbation (a period of worsened symptoms, usually due to a respiratory infection), contracting pneumonia, going downhill, and losing ground, never fully recovering to where they were.

As a person with COPD, your job is to be on the look-out for early warning signs of acute exacerbation. A

cold or flu germ that is a mere inconvenience to someone with healthy lungs can become a major problem for
you, possibly leading to something serious. But there are
things you can do to stave off an acute exacerbation of
COPD. This is not to say you'll be completely successful
at doing so each and every time, but if you know what
to avoid and what signs to watch for, you'll be in a much
better position to minimize illness and keep on living
your life.

Avoiding germs

Below are just a few of the many things you can do to
avoid picking up nasty bugs. I'm sure you can think of
others that work well for you:

* Get your flu shot every fall.
* Get a pneumonia shot every five to seven years
  depending on your doctor's recommendation.
* Wash your hands with warm water and mild
  soap. Wash for fifteen seconds – the time it takes
  to sing "Twinkle, Twinkle Little Star." (You don't
  have to sing aloud!)
* Use your own pen. Do you really want to touch
  that pen (the one everybody uses) at the bank – or
  worse yet, the doctor's office?
* If you can't wipe it off, wear lightweight gloves
  or cover the handle of the grocery cart when you
  shop.
* Carry hand sanitizer with you and use it when
  you can't wash.

Develop an action plan with your doctor

Work in partnership with your doctor to stay well. Make
an appointment if you don't have one coming up soon.
At this appointment, ask:

* "When do you want me to call you?"
* "Which early warning signs do you want to know about when I notice them?"
* "When I call your office, how will your staff know that I'm more likely than many of your other patients to get really sick?"

Know what to watch for

Knowing early warning signs cannot only help you stay healthy, at home and independent, but it can even save your life! Here are some early warning signs of acute exacerbation for people with COPD. Show this list to your doctor and ask if there are any other early warning signs, specific to you and your situation, that he or she suggests you watch for.

* A change in your cough – are you coughing more, less, or is it different than usual?
* A change in the amount, color, or texture of your sputum (Yes, you should be looking at it!). Is it yellow, green, or bloody? Is it thick or sticky? Your mucous should be thin and clear or white.
* If you have a pulse oximeter at home, are your O2 sats (oxygen saturations) lower than usual?
* Sudden weight gain such as 3-5 lbs. overnight.
* Swelling in your ankles or feet. Here's a tip: Gently press the tip of your finger into the skin around your ankles and feet. Does it leave a dent? It shouldn't. If it does, call your doctor.
* Morning dizziness, confusion, or headache that doesn't go away with medications such as Tylenol or Advil.
* A heart rate faster than usual (60-100 is normal with each person having their own "normal"). Know your normal resting heart rate.

* Your urine should be pale yellow and clear, with no odor. If it is darker or cloudy, or with a foul odor, you might have a urinary tract infection.
* Fever.
* Unusual fatigue.
* Joint or muscle aches.

Don't spend this fall and winter on the edge of a COPD exacerbation! If you catch early warning signs and work in partnership with your doctor, you have a much better chance at stopping an infection in its tracks, so you can stay well and get on with living.

Your Turn

Key points, or … If you don't remember anything else from this chapter, remember this:

- As a person with COPD you can, and must:
- Do what you can to avoid lung infections.
- Know the early warning signs of acute exacerbation.
- Develop an action plan with your doctor about when to call and how to make sure the office staff is alert to your needs.

Ask yourself this:

- Do I know the early warning signs of acute exacerbation?

This week:

- Make an appointment with your doctor for a flu shot and a discussion of how to stay healthy this fall and winter.

Here's more help

- There are two copies of "Early Warning Signs" in this book, one at the end of this chapter and the other at the end of this book. If this is your own copy of *Live Your Life with COPD*, tear out the page, bring it to your next appointment, show it to your doctor and ask him or her to help you complete it. Then keep it where you can see it, as a reminder to do all you can to stay healthy this fall and winter."

Early Warning Signs of Acute Exacerbation of COPD

* A change in your cough – are you coughing more, less, or is it different than usual?
* A change in the amount or color of your sputum. Is it yellow, green, or bloody? Your mucous should be clear or white.
* If you have a pulse oximeter at home, are your O2 sats (oxygen saturations) lower than usual?
* Sudden weight gain such as 3-5 lbs. overnight.
* Swelling in your ankles or feet. Here's a tip: Gently press the tip of your finger into the skin around your ankles and feet. Does it leave a dent? It shouldn't. If it does, call your doctor.
* Morning dizziness, confusion, or headache that doesn't go away with medications such as Tylenol or Advil.
* A heart rate faster than usual (60-100 is normal with each person having their own "normal"). Know your normal resting heart rate.
* Your urine should be pale yellow and clear, with no odor. If it is darker than usual, cloudy, or with a foul odor, you might have a urinary tract infection.
* Fever.
* Unusual fatigue.
* Joint or muscle aches.
• Other_____
  _____
  _____

(over)

My Exacerbation Prevention Plan:

_____

_____

_____

_____

_____

_____

Dr. _____

Office phone number: _____

Cough and Airway Clearance
[JMM]

You gotta do what you gotta do.
– Sylvester Stallone

Phlegm. Secretions. Sputum. Mucous. Yuck! Whatever you call it, that junk in your lungs is yet another part of having COPD that's not a lot of fun. Yet, it's one of those things that as a person with COPD, you just have to deal with – and if you learn what to expect and how to handle it, you'll breathe easier.

What's the role of sputum in the lungs?

Before we talk about getting rid of secretions, we need to understand why we have them in the first place.

The lungs provide protection against foreign substances entering the body by stopping unwanted particles and trapping them before they get too deep into your lungs. Lining the airways inside your lungs (the breathing tubes, bronchi and bronchioles that carry the air) is a mucous blanket, a thin layer of mucous. Just underneath this mucous blanket are cilia, millions of tiny little hair-like structures. The cilia move like a wave to help propel the mucous – carrying with it trapped dust, bacteria, and other substances upward, where they can be coughed out. This is how your lungs keep themselves clean.

Mucous also acts to humidify the air you breathe. As your air makes its way through your bronchial tubes, it passes over the mucous, picking up moisture.

You may be wondering why people with healthy lungs don't cough routinely. The answer is that they probably do, coughing a minimal amount of sputum up and out, or swallowing (and digesting) it. In healthy lungs mucous is rarely a problem so it goes unnoticed.

Dirty lungs

Remember the cilia, the little sweepers in your airways that help keep your lungs clean? Cigarette smoke and other irritants in our environment can destroy or paralyze them. This causes the cilia to stop functioning and thus, your lungs are not able to clean themselves as they should. Along with this the breathing tubes can become chronically (continually) or acutely (suddenly and temporarily) swollen and inflamed. As a result, the airways may produce thicker and stickier mucous secretions.

With the loss of your normal cleaning mechanism as well as a tendency towards thicker, stickier secretions and swollen airways, you can see why breathing with COPD can be so difficult! With all this going on, your lungs are left to figure out another way to get rid of excess mucous and that's why you may have a frequent, productive cough. If you cough on most days, producing sputum, even when you do not have an acute infection, you probably have chronic bronchitis. Ask your doctor to be sure.

All of this sticky mucous can make it difficult to breathe, but there's another reason why it's important to keep your lungs clear. If sputum is not cleared from the lungs, it can cause ongoing inflammation, which can lead to further lung damage – and more coughing – making you tired and even more breathless.

What can I do to keep my lungs clear?

* Take time – make time – for bronchial hygiene (keeping your lungs clean and clear) each day, just as you take time to wash your face or brush your teeth.
* Drink two quarts of water a day, if approved by your doctor.
* Take an expectorant or mucolytic, if necessary. This can be ordered by your doctor, or you can take a non-prescription expectorant if your doctor says it's okay.
* Use proper cough technique. Sit up straight, but bending slightly forward with elbow support. A straight chair with armrests works well.
* If at all possible, do not lie down when coughing. Coughing is much more effective when sitting up.
* Use the huff cough technique. Ask a respiratory therapist to show you.
* Ask your doctor if Percussion and Postural Drainage might help. If so, a respiratory therapist can train your family member or caregiver how to perform this therapy.
* Use an airway clearance device if directed (see below).

Below is a report on Mucous Clearance Devices contributed by Richard D. Martin, the Editor of *COPD-NEWS*. Thank you to Richard for authorizing the reprint of this information.

In some cases, our doctors or respiratory therapists might recommend we use a hand-held mechanism that loosens the mucous to make it easier to cough out. These small devices vibrate when we breathe into them and are known by various names, such as "percussive airway devices," or "vibratory positive expiratory pressure (PEP) devices." They use vibrations and air pressure to reduce the thickness of mucous. Although the devices are used more commonly for individuals with Cystic Fibrosis and bronchiectasis, they are also used to help those of us with COPD who have difficulty getting rid of mucous.

There are a number of brands on the market. They all require a prescription. The most commonly recognized brands are Acapella, Flutter, Lung Flute, and Quake, although there are others. Your doctor or respiratory therapist may recommend a particular brand for a specific reason. In some cases, they actually keep a small supply on hand and dispense them directly to patients. It pays, however, to be familiar with the major brands.

If you are prescribed a device, be sure to have a respiratory therapist teach you how to use it properly. It may seem simple, but there is more to it than just blowing into it!

(This information is current as of late 2010. For more information, use an Internet search engine, typing in the name of the device along with the words, "Airway Clearance," or ask your respiratory health professional.)

Acapella

This device shakes your mucous loose when you blow into it. It must be dialed to the proper setting by someone who is trained in its use. It will work if you are lying down.

Flutter

The Flutter works in a similar way, but you must be sitting or standing up straight to use it.

Lung Flute

The Flute creates vibrations to loosen the mucus by passing air over a reed. The device includes a six-month supply of reeds. An additional six month supply must be purchased.

Quake

The Quake works on both inspiratory and expiratory phases of breathing.

Bonus Box
When Coughing is Too Distasteful
A lifetime of suppression leads to infection – and a very unladylike treatment for Lady Windermere Syndrome.

By Francis V. Adams, Special to *The Los Angeles Times,* March 26, 2007.

Coughing was a no-no for a proper lady. (Columbia Pictures)

I saw another Lady Windermere the other day. Over the years I have seen several patients who could have borne this name. The character originated in Oscar Wilde's play "Lady Windermere's Fan." She was a fastidious woman who at one moment refuses to shake hands with a visitor ("My hands are all wet with the roses"). Wilde's character would become a symbol of the Victorian era, an age when women wouldn't do anything they thought vulgar, such as spitting.

My first Lady Windermere was Agatha. I met her not long after I finished my training in pulmonary disease and opened my private practice. I glimpsed her in the waiting room as I picked up her chart. A few minutes later, as she sat in my office, I inquired as to what had brought her, and she went on to describe an unrelenting cough she'd had for nearly 10 years. During the interview, she coughed fitfully but would not expectorate.

Agatha was 63, very thin, almost skeletal, with high cheekbones, thin lips and a straight nose. Her forehead was made more prominent by her graying hair, which was pulled straight back. She held a tiny lace handkerchief in her left hand and covered her mouth as she coughed.

I proceeded to take Agatha's medical history. She had been in good health except for her chest problems, which she described as frequent colds that always settled in her chest. Agatha had been hospitalized twice for pneumonia. She was an actress and had done stage and film, mostly small parts as she described them. Agatha's physical examination did not add much to what I had already observed. Her lung sounds were a bit quieter than normal but I did not detect any congestion. I proceeded to take an X-ray, which showed that the air passages in the middle sections were thicker than normal.

We sat in my office and I told her that it would help if she could bring up some sputum for the lab to analyze for infection. I also explained that additional X-rays would be helpful.

The culture of the tiny piece of expectorated sputum yielded an organism known as mycobacterium avium intracellulare. This is a ubiquitous germ that lives in nature and can be found in the soil or water. At this point in my practice, I had seen this infection only in immune- compromised individuals but knew it could occur in anyone with damaged lungs. Agatha had no history of childhood infection so I wondered if the over-fastidiousness that kept her from clearing secretions had in fact promoted the development of her condition. I proceeded to outline a course of treatment that would include three antibiotics over a period of one-and-a-half years. I also placed her on an expectorant and arranged for a physical therapist to cup and clap her chest twice a week, hoping to help clear her air passages. Despite these efforts, my patient's cough did not produce sputum.

During the long course of Agatha's treatment, I saw two more women who bore not only a physical resemblance to her but also the identical illness. Irene was 68, a teacher with a widow's peak, and Constance was 60, a librarian. Both had similar X-ray changes as Agatha, and their sputum, which I obtained with great difficulty, also yielded the same organism. All three women were cooperative, intelligent, and easy to work with, but I became increasingly frustrated by their failure to clear their lungs despite the many maneuvers that I put them through.

After my third case, I consulted my colleagues and the medical literature and found that I was not alone.

Other doctors were seeing similar patients. In 1992, 15 years after I first met Agatha, two radiologists published a report of "The Lady Windermere Syndrome." They had observed six women with the same characteristics as my patients. The authors noted that the middle portions of the lungs extend outward toward the front of the chest and require vigorous coughing for clearance of secretions. They concluded that mycobacterial infection had occurred in these overly fastidious women due to voluntary suppression of cough.

In the last several years, greater numbers of cases of mycobacterial infection have been reported. Unfortunately the treatment is not always successful and may be difficult to tolerate due to adverse effects of the antibiotics.

Agatha's infection was not cured by years of treatment but did improve. I continue to see a few women each year with the same striking features and pride myself on making the correct diagnosis simply from observing their appearance and hearing their cough before they are seated in my office.

A few of these delicate women have found me through Internet searches so that after introducing myself to one of these ladies recently, she replied: "And you may call me Lady Windermere."

Reprinted with permission from Dr. Francis V. Adams. Dr. Adams is a pulmonologist in New York City and the author of *The Asthma Sourcebook 3rd Edition*, *The Breathing Disorders Sourcebook*, and *Healing Through Empathy-An Expanded Edition.*

Your Turn

Key points, or … If you don't remember anything else from this chapter, remember this:

- Lungs have a built-in cleaning system that can be impaired or disabled with COPD.
- It's important to do all you can to keep your lungs clear, not only for good health now, but to protect your lungs from further damage.
- There are many things you can do to help clear your lungs.
- Practice bronchial hygiene every day – not just when you're having problems.

Ask yourself this:

- Do I cough every day?
- Do I bring up mucous?
- Do I have trouble bringing up mucous, feeling like it's "stuck"?

This week:

- If you answer "yes" to any of the three questions above, make sure you're taking all the steps in "What Can I Do to Keep My Lungs Clear?"
- Go back and read this chapter at least one more time this week.

Here's more help

- COPD News http://copd-support.com/news.html

Denial
[JMM]

The worst lies are the lies we tell ourselves.
– Richard Bach

When I was researching for my first book, interviewing people with COPD – people from all walks of life, of all ages, from all over the country – I found that without exception there was one common thread connecting every story. Denial. Let's be honest, no one wants to even think of having an incurable, progressive disease, especially one that may have been brought on by a particular behavior. We're all human and we like to think of ourselves as being active and healthy. So of course, denial is extremely common in COPD.

This book is about COPD, and I am assuming that you, the reader, already know – or strongly suspect – that you have this disease. But, in this chapter we're going to turn the clock back and talk about that period of time, probably a period of years, in which you didn't know you had COPD. A time when you first maybe, barely, noticed shortness of breath. And we're going to retrace your steps all the way up to that pivotal moment or event when finally, it was undeniable.

Small changes – What changes?

We're all getting older, and along with advancing age we can expect to slow down. Becoming short of breath is probably one of the most common small changes we experience – and one of the easiest to pass over as insignificant.

Cheri Register is the author of *The Chronic Illness Experience*. Although Cheri has a non-pulmonary related chronic disease, we can learn a lot from her experience. She says, "The first challenge any illness poses is in deciding just when you are sick enough to worry about it. Often the initial problems are not that great a departure from your usual state of health. As annoying as they might be, you may be tempted to dismiss them, unless they are known to be danger signals, like the (more well-known) 'warning signs of cancer.' Everyone has aches and pains, after all, and most of them subside on their own. For fear of being called hypochondriacs, many of us would rather wait out the discomfort than risk seeming excessively alarmed."

Gradual Changes – or – "Maybe if I just ignore it, it'll go away."

When I asked Mary Pierce (a lady with Alpha-1 COPD – see chapter April -Week 1) if she thought her husband, Todd, knew something was wrong, Mary answered, "He says he didn't. When people later on asked him, 'Didn't you know that something was going on?' He answered, 'Well, I knew she was losing a lot of weight, but it just happened so gradually, I never noticed [the increasing shortness of breath].' Because, again, he was making all the little incremental adjustments along the way."

Cheri Register's take on it: "It is not so much fear and denial as it is confusion and embarrassment that keep people out of the doctor's office in the early stages of illness. Having no clear sense of the boundaries that divide illness from health, we redraw our own as needed, to keep ourselves functioning."

Whatever we call it – fear, denial, confusion, embarrassment – though chronic lung disease symptoms may temporarily subside, they eventually demand attention.

I was just fine until...

It's important to understand that in all but a few cases, by the time you seek help, your COPD has been progressing for quite some time, probably for years or even decades. A classic scenario is the patient states that he or she was just fine until recently coming down with pneumonia. Upon further examination (Chest X-ray, Pulmonary Function, Arterial Blood Gas, and personal health history) it becomes abundantly clear to the doctor and, eventually to the patient, that lung disease has been present for many years.

As the lungs become more and more compromised over time they are less able to tolerate common insults such as colds and flu. What a shock to the person who feels they were fine until a recent illness, and is now told they have 30% lung function left (70% non-functional and beyond repair)!

A pulmonary doctor reminds us, "One day you walk up to your car and notice a spot of rust. You never noticed it before. You're sure it wasn't there yesterday. And it probably wasn't. But, do you think that until today the body of your car in that spot was perfectly intact? It was solid, perfect metal and then, overnight, it broke through to form a rusty patch? No, you see the rust and realize then that it must have been coming on for quite a while."

Significant event – the tipping point

It's been said that denial is nature's way of giving us a good night's sleep. Maybe so, but this works only up to a point; and especially with COPD, there often comes a time when there are simply no more excuses, no more denying the facts.

When I interview new patients coming into the pulmonary rehab program, one of the first questions I ask is when did they first notice their shortness of breath? Almost always, they tell me of a point in time, something they remember well, a moment that tipped the scale causing them to sit up and take note that something is not only not right, but something is very wrong.

Cheri Register sheds some light on this. "We continue to tell these stories [of when the illness began] because it seems important to have a frame in which to contain the experience of chronic illness. The story needs a strong beginning because it has no structure otherwise. With chronic illness, there is no single climax, just the irregularly recurring ups and downs... Chronic illness does not fit the popular notion of how illness proceeds: 'You get sick, you go to the doctor and get some medicine, and wait to get better'... The best we can do to clear up the chaos in our lives is to look back and say, 'This is how it all began. This was when my life took an unfortunate turn.'"

Going way back

Back to the pulmonary rehab initial evaluation – as we talk, we delve a bit deeper, and as we do, the patient thinks back to times *before* the turning point, often saying, "Now that I think about it, I remember several years ago having some trouble keeping up. I figured I was getting older and out of shape, so I didn't think much of it."

Guilt and Shame

Mary Pierce (a former smoker with Alpha-1 Antitrypsin Deficiency, genetically inherited COPD) said of her life before diagnosis, "The denial was definitely there... for a *long* time. It was like I was the only one who had *the secret*... a huge dark secret. The hiding. The shame. The guilt... You know, I'd seen other people with health problems worse than mine, things they didn't bring on themselves. I figured, by smoking, I'd shortened my life and all that. *I did it to myself.* At the time I didn't think it all the way through, but my reaction then was guilt, shame, embarrassment."

Relationships – With your family

Mary continues, "At least I felt that way, and I was hiding it from everybody. I was denying it and hiding it, and that was part of who I was. That alone prevented some of the close personal interactions…the wall was up, even with my family. The interactions became artificial. You know, pretending…I remember back when I could not do much of anything. I just didn't have the energy. I'd say, 'I can't. I've got to go do this or I've got to do that.' I'd just make an excuse somehow."

Relationships – With your doctor

Denial can also adversely affect your relationship with your physician. There can be no partnership in effective lung health management if the doctor is unaware of your breathing problems.

Consequently, without the right information, it's not possible to make informed end-of-life decisions regarding life support, or "heroic" measures. More than anyone, the person with chronic disease needs to discuss end-of-life issues with family in order to make informed decisions together. The decisions must be written down and placed where medical personnel and family can easily find them. Not doing so, puts a burden on family members who are faced not only with making difficult decisions in a time of crisis, but need to make those decisions in light of a chronic diagnosis that to them – because of denial – seems so new.

In some cases the diagnosis has been given, but under-stated by the doctor. Some patients are told by their doctor that they have a "little touch" of emphysema. This might even be considered denial on the part of the physician!

Mary Pierce says, "Those words 'a little touch' kind of put the patient on notice that they don't have to worry about it. Hearing a wishy-washy diagnosis is like going into confessional and being forgiven."

Poor Health Management

With denial, there is no diagnosis. With no diagnosis, there is no effective management, and one's overall health will only get worse. Denial of the existence of COPD can actually lead to a person obtaining either less – or sur-prisingly more – treatment than needed. Treating each exacerbation as an isolated case, as just another "bout of bronchitis," can cause over-prescribing of antibiot-ics. Failure to treat COPD symptoms at all, on the other hand, denies the patient the opportunity to benefit from helpful medications, education, support, and exercise that can extend and improve the quality of life.

Does this mean I'm giving in? And does it mean I'm giving up?

Finally, and so importantly, just because you admit and accept the diagnosis of chronic lung disease does not mean you're about to give up. Far from it! Acceptance gives you the permission and the *power* to acquire knowl-edge – knowledge that will arm you with weapons needed for the battle to fight your disease. With the help of a good physician, and referral to a pulmonary specialist and a Pulmonary Rehabilitation Program if possible, you can begin the process of breathing better and living well.

Traveling the road from denial to acceptance and empowerment can be a long, painful journey. But when you know what you're facing, you can find help. With the support of knowledgeable respiratory health professionals, understanding peers, and a loving family, you can learn what works and what doesn't, what is achievable and what isn't, what is realistic and what is no longer safe to attempt. Finally, free from the grip of denial, you can gain control of your breathing with hope for the best possible life from that moment on.

Bonus Box

Meet Tom, a successful businessman with a drive to work hard and keep on going, no matter what. Here, in his own words, he gives us a glimpse of a fascinating timeline on his road to better breathing.

Let me start with a few flash backs that seem to make sense now. 1974 – Age 31. I didn't have any problems. We were moving into a new house and my father, a healthy non-smoker of 71, was helping me carry things. After moving one particularly heavy desk a relatively short distance he was left gasping for air. I never thought much of this until recently. He was never diagnosed with a breathing disorder. He died of congestive heart failure four years later.

1982 – Age 39. I didn't have any problems. We were skiing. A big snow fell and we were out first thing in of my the morning. I made a run to the bottom and fell in a heap. After catching my breath I tried to get up but the snow was too deep and I just wallowed around. It took me ten minutes of struggling and resting to finally get back to my feet. I thought I was going to faint.

1997 – Age 54. I didn't have any problems. I was at one of my daughter's high school basketball games – a championship at stake. A see-saw game with the crowd going wild. All of a sudden I realized that after a cheer I had nothing left in my lungs. Gulp, gulp, a little air, please.

2007 – Age 63. I checked in with a pulmonologist who sent me over to the hospital for testing. Sure enough, I was operating with less than 40% expected lung capacity. He had suggestions about how I could manage my disease. But, of course, things got in the way and I put it off.

2008 – Age 64. I was standing in the grocery store gasping for breath. I had an infection, my lungs were full of liquid, and I flat out couldn't breathe.

And so I entered Pulmonary Rehabilitation.

I guess my first thought when I was clearly told and shown the hard data proving that I had COPD was, "Well, let's get to work fixing this mess." I am a pretty hard-nosed realist and have spent my life in design and problem solving, so this was nothing new. I also reflected on the fact that I had a good idea of what it is that will kill me.

My first thought at starting pulmonary rehab was, "Wow, I'm in far better shape than everyone else here... I'm lucky to have this chance, and I had better take it seriously and bust my butt to get in shape."

My daily life is just as it has been these last ten years, except I am in rehab for two hours a week, I lift weights for two hours a week, I have learned how to do purse-lipped breathing, and I plan ahead and start breathing early when I know I'm headed for some stairs. You have to commit the time and – given the alternative – that should be easy.

I guess I was in denial for a long time. Certainly long enough! But now, after facing COPD head on, learning about it, and doing all I can to manage it, I have to tell you – my Quality of Life is better, and I have no doubt that my *Quantity of Life* will be better, too.

Your Turn

Key points, or ... If you don't remember anything else from this chapter, remember this:

- Getting past denial is an essential step in becoming empowered to live life to the fullest with COPD.

Ask yourself this:

- Where am I in this process?

This week:

- Write the timeline of your own journey from denial to empowerment.

Here's more help

- "Take Back Your Life Framework," chapter May – Week 1

Advance Directives
Why You (and Everyone) Should Have a Living Will
[JMM]

*Having the world's best idea will do you no good
unless you act on it.
People who want milk shouldn't sit on a stool in the
middle of a field in hopes that a cow will back up to them.*
– Curtis Grant

Dr. Rajani, a tiny lady no more than five feet tall, shook my hand, looked me in the eye and said, "Your father is a very sick man. His body is shutting down. Do you want us to put him on life support or should we make him a 'no code'?"

"Uh…can we watch him closely and see…"

She interrupted. "You have to make a decision. Soon."

Not exactly what I had in mind for my first meeting with this doctor and certainly not the best way to begin a discussion on end-of-life issues!

My sister had called me the night before saying that Dad was in the hospital in Chicago with shortness of breath, but after getting settled in and being put on oxygen, he was feeling more comfortable and doing better. The next morning, however, mom called me at my hospital job in Michigan, saying, "Dad's taken a turn for the worse and they say he might not make it." Her voice wavered. "I need you here. You understand these things."

You see, as Dad got older, my sister and I had urged him to talk about what he would prefer be done, medically, if he were unable to speak for himself. But, stubborn Dutchman that he was (eighty years old at the time and more obstinate than ever), he refused. Now, here we were. Inaction on my father's part had put all of us – my mom, the doctors, my sister, and me – in this terrible, and most urgent, situation. Believe me, you don't want to find yourself in this position – and the good news is you don't ever have to. Let's talk about advance directives, appointing a patient advocate, and living wills.

What is an Advance Directive?

An advance directive is a document – made in advance – detailing what you would like done if you should be unable to speak for yourself in a medical situation. An advance directive allows you to make your own decisions, and by doing so, maintain control over what happens to you so others don't make decisions for you. Telling your loved ones your wishes is a good first step, but it is not enough. You must have it in writing.

What is a Living Will?

A living will is a legal document in which you make your wishes known regarding life-prolonging medical treatments. A living will should not be confused with a living trust, which has to do with holding and distributing your property and finances.

Who should have one?

Every adult should have a living will, even those who are young and healthy.

What is a Durable Power of Attorney for Health Care?

This is the appointment of a patient advocate; one or two people you have chosen to speak for you if you should ever be unable to speak for yourself. This could be a spouse, an adult child, or someone else you trust who is able, and willing, to take responsibility for carrying out your wishes.

How do I start this discussion? Isn't it morbid and depressing? Will it scare my loved ones?

No one likes to think about dying or losing a loved one, but we are all going to die sometime, and when we do, it should be on our own terms. Begin by assuring your loved ones that bringing up this subject doesn't mean you're planning to die anytime soon. Take a positive approach – assure them you're doing this to maintain your dignity and ensure your wishes are implemented. Remind them as well, that if this time should come it would be much easier on them if your instructions were known in advance.

Should I talk about this with my doctor?

Yes! Bring it up at your next appointment, or make a special appointment for this purpose. It's shocking to know that one study revealed that 83% of patients with advanced COPD had not discussed end-of-life wishes with their physician, although 78% said they wanted to[6]. Talk honestly with your doctor about options that are right for you and the state of your disease.

How do I get started?

Your local hospital should have forms that are legal in your state, and they should have a social worker or nurse

6. Michel Chalhoub, MD, Staten Island University Hospital in New York, presented findings to the annual meeting of the American College of Chest Physicians, 2003, Orlando, Florida.

to assist you. A lawyer can also help you. There are many resources on the Internet. Just make sure that documents are legal in your state, as laws vary from state to state. The charge for downloading or sending for such documents should be modest. There are many good ones costing no more than $30.00.

You might be wondering what happened with Dad. Well, after ten days in the ICU, he pulled through and lived for nearly two more years. He was well enough in that time to see grandchildren get married and graduate from college and high school – and he even went back to work part time. Also during that time he made it clear to all of us exactly what he wanted should he ever get that sick again and be unable to speak for himself. Finally, when he had no fight left in him, he passed away quietly with no tubes, no machines, and no pain – with family at his side. Yes, it took a while for a proud man to talk about end-of-life care, but we're so glad he did.

Your Turn

Key points, or... If you don't remember anything else from this chapter, remember this:

- Everybody should have an advance directive.
- Preparing an advance directive in writing assures you that your wishes (not the wishes or assumptions of others) will be carried out if you are ever unable to speak for yourself.
- You should talk with your doctor about end-of-life issues.
- Completing a legal advance directive can be easy and inexpensive.

Ask yourself this:

- Do I have the two parts of an Advance Directive: Durable Power of Attorney for Healthcare and a Living Will?
- Do you know where it is?
- Do your advocates have copies?
- Is it due to be updated?

This week:

- If you don't have an advance directive, talk with your loved ones about it.
- If you do have an advance directive, be proud that you have that out of the way, so go out and do something fun that has to do with *living* – not dying!

Here's more help

- Legacy Writer https://www.legacywriter.com/
- Legal Zoom http://www.legalzoom.com/sem/livingwillpage.html
- Call your local hospital or physician's office for information and forms that are legal in your state. Many times these are free of charge.

Depression
[JMM]

Never despair.
– Horace

"I'm fighting for every breath here, doc. I can't do anything I used to. I was a strong guy – a firefighter for goodness sake. Now I can barely carry my garden hose! I can't sleep, I can't concentrate, I don't feel like doing anything anymore." Jerry sat across from Dr. Rogers and leaned forward with his elbows on his knees. He looked down and sighed. "I don't know, doc. This COPD thing has really knocked me down."

Jerry is experiencing a few of the many signs of clinical depression, and he's not alone. Depression is common in people with COPD. And why shouldn't it be? After all, it's like any other chronic disease, right? Well, maybe not. Experts are learning more about depression in people with COPD, and they're finding that there may be an even closer connection than we thought[7].

To start, let's take a quick look at COPD and how it can affect your emotional well-being. Left untreated, COPD can be a wasting disease. You begin to do less and less, becoming increasingly weak until you're unable to do much of anything at all. This can lead to diminished independence prompting feelings of anger, frustration, isolation and loss of control. Once

7. "The risk for depression comorbidity in patients with COPD."
Published online before print August 8, 2008, doi: 10.1378/chest.08-0965
http://www.chestjournal.org/conent/early/2008//08/08/chest.08-0965.
abstract

you're on this downward spiral, depression may not be far behind.

How do you know if you might be depressed?

What are the symptoms of depression?

* Loss of interest in favorite activities
* Always tired
* Frequent sadness
* Irritability
* Significant weight change
* Wishing to be left alone
* Hopelessness
* Trouble sleeping
* Lack of appetite
* Thoughts of death or suicide
* Feeling worthless or guilty for no reason
* Difficulty concentrating

If you feel this way, or are even beginning to feel this way, you may be heading for depression. If any of these symptoms start to creep up on you, take action!

What should you do?

* Tell your doctor if you have any of these symptoms.
* Ask him or her about anti-depressant medication and if this might be appropriate for you.
* Ask your doctor if you should talk with a counselor or other mental health specialist. It is not a sign of weakness to talk with someone about issues that affect your happiness and well-being. Really.
* Ask your doctor to refer you to Pulmonary Rehabilitation (see chapter January – Week 5). There you will learn how to exercise, safely and

effectively – even if you're very short of breath. This will help you build up your strength and use your oxygen more efficiently. The more fit you are, the more confidence you have, and the more your outlook improves. At pulmonary rehab you'll learn tips for staying healthy – and you'll meet others who understand what it's like to live each day with COPD.

* Talk with an understanding friend or clergy. Sometimes just sitting down and talking about what you're going through can make your problems easier to deal with.
* Give yourself a change of scenery by taking a walk or drive. Just getting out of the house can help you feel much better. Seeing something new helps take your mind off yourself. If possible, make it a routine to get out of the house at least three times a week.
* Join a group – a breathing support group or one based on a hobby – book club, stamp collecting, quilting, something that makes you feel good. The wider you can make your circle of acquaintances, the better.
* Educate your family. As well-intentioned as your loved ones may be, they often have no idea what it's like to live with COPD.
* Help others by volunteering. Even with shortness of breath, there are things you can do to make your community a better place. Check with your local hospital, school, house of worship, or library, to ask what you can do.

So, what did Dr. Rogers say?

"Jerry, it sounds like you're depressed. I think we can help you with that."

"Oh, I don't know… Maybe I'm just getting old."

"This happens to a lot of folks. I'm going to send you over to see Lynda, the respiratory therapist at pulmonary rehab. She can tell you about the program. I think you could also benefit from talking with someone about this."

"Now, wait a minute, doc… I'm not going to a shrink. I'll just give myself a kick and I'll be fine."

Dr. Rogers smiled. "Okay, no 'shrink,' for now. How about your pastor? I'll bet he'd be happy to take a few minutes to sit down and talk with you."

"Well, he's always asking me to stop over for coffee…"

"Good. You give him a call. Today. And one more thing – I'm giving you a prescription for an anti-depressant.

"Hold on now… I've never been one to…"

"Just give it a try, and if you don't think it's working, let me know. But, I really think it'll help." He paused. "Okay, Jerry, are you all set? Anything else you want to ask me?"

"Nope, I think that's it, doc. Thanks."

Depression is common in people with COPD. But it's nothing to be ashamed of! Watch for the signs of depression. Recognize them, accept them for what they are, talk to your doctor, and then follow through with the help that's available. Beware of that nasty monster – depression. He'll sneak up on you if you let him. But now that you know who he is and what to do, you can fight him off – and get on with living.

Your Turn

Key points, or . . . If you don't remember anything else from this chapter, remember this:

- Depression is common in people with COPD.
- Being depressed does not mean you are weak-minded.
- Depression can be treated effectively in a variety of ways.
- It's important to watch for signs of depression and know that although well-controlled at one time, may manifest again.

Ask yourself this:

- Do I have any symptoms of depression?

This week:

- If you have symptoms of depression, make an appointment, today, with your doctor to talk about it.

Here's more help

- *The Mindfulness & Acceptance Workbook for Depression: Using Acceptance & Commitment Therapy to Move Through Depression & Create a Life Worth Living,* by Kirk D. Strosahl, PH.D. and Patricia J. Robinson, PH.D.
- National Jewish Health – COPD Emotional Management:
  http://www.nationaljewish.org/healthinfo/conditions/copd/emotional-management/index.aspx

Additional Therapies for COPD
Massage, Yoga, and Tai Chi
[JMM]

When you're through changing, you're through.
– Bruce Barton

When learning about living well with COPD, of course we should focus on the basics of good lung health, such as medications, nutrition, breathing techniques, and exercise, etc. It's also important – essential, in fact – to pay close attention to emotional issues, such as anxiety, denial, and relationships, to name a few. But in this chapter we're going to talk about some other forms of therapy that can help you stay healthy with COPD, things you might never have thought could have a positive effect on your breathing. These are Yoga, Tai Chi, and Massage.

Elsewhere in this book you'll find references to yoga and tai chi. In Chapter July – Week 3 Relaxation, Dr. Sharma provides a step-by-step routine for relaxation and breathing relating to yoga techniques. Jo-Von Tucker talks briefly about the benefits of tai chi in Chapter April – Week 4 – Coping with Stress. And in this chapter you'll find the personal story of a lady with severe COPD who discovered the benefits of massage.

If you think massage might help you, ask your doctor or lung health professional if it would be safe for you to try. Understand that things like yoga, tai chi and massage are not meant to replace the treatment program prescribed by your doctor, but to enhance it. Always consult your doctor before starting any new therapy.

Ask around and talk with people who have had this particular treatment.

As always, when you have a chronic medical condition, be sure you're working with people who have:
* Accreditation and experience in their discipline
* A willingness to provide references
* Experience working specifically with people with COPD

Below is one lady's experience with massage and how it affected her life with COPD. I know you'll find it interesting – and inspiring.

A classmate of mine in pulmonary rehab maintenance mentioned one day that she was getting massage for pain issues. She said that she felt so much better and also that she felt she could breathe better. And I could see that she did. She recommended I consider massage for myself and she gave me the number of her massage therapist. So, skeptical as I was, I trusted my rehab friend and made an appointment with Terri.

I have to tell you…I'm not one of *those* women who go in for "spa days" and what I consider the primping sort of things. That's what I always thought massage was – like manicures and pedicures. Things that are okay to do, but I thought, a waste of good money. I mean, I would rather buy a pair of shoes, or a something for my grandson, or go out to lunch with a friend – anything but "waste" the money on myself!

Another reason I was hesitant to have a massage was my own vanity. I've lost so much weight and as you may know, the skin just doesn't shrink as we age!

People think of me as being tiny. I'm 5'2" and weigh 97 pounds. One girl joked at pulmonary rehab that she was *born* larger than I am now! Others say I am so thin I might break! This is just my body, so I am not really aware of what they're referring to. On the other hand, I don't think others can picture me as I see myself – with saggy skin from severe weight loss, the wrinkles and scars left by surgeries, and all of that. I used to be pretty strong – muscular to a point – well-toned and proud of how I looked in a bikini! No way, now! I was so worried about someone seeing "all of me" in my newer shrunken state; I couldn't embarrass myself!

But when the day came, I found the courage and went ahead and kept my appointment. I found out that my Massage Therapist has a nursing background and I think that is one thing that makes her so effective for someone with severe COPD like mine (I am down to around 19-20% FEV_1, so that is quite an issue for me).

I was relieved, also, to find out that in massage the therapist only uncovers whatever part she is working on and never sees me completely undressed! If I had known that I might have gone sooner!

You might be concerned that during massage you'd have to lie down on a flat surface. Some people with COPD can't lie flat and need to have their head raised a bit. If this is the case, you can ask your massage therapist if he or she can work around that. I cannot go from moving around a lot, being winded, and then just lying down flat. But I can do it, if I do it in stages.

Another issue I was concerned about was the cost. Just how much was this luxury going to cost me? Well, if I were still smoking it would be about a trade-off with a carton of cigs. Maybe a tiny bit more, but oh, so beneficial!

I've now gone five weeks in a row, and even my husband is impressed with how much better I'm doing. At the first session, I talked my way through it – telling Terri about all my pain and what had caused it (surgeries and other injuries). The second time she had to wake me up. I gave in to just relaxing to the feel of her hands and the background music. The last few sessions have been a combination.

Undeniably, I am breathing better and I am so much more relaxed. The tension she has been able to release from my muscles is amazing. I was just so tightened up I'm surprised I was able to breathe at all!

I would highly recommend considering massage therapy to anyone, whether you're a man or a woman, with tension build-up, breathing issues, pain issues, or just in need of a "self-preservation" experience. I can state that it was, and will continue to be, well worth the expenditure for me! Ask around for a good referral. Not all therapists are alike and word does get around about a good one. They're here to help and appreciate knowing their clients referred them. Wouldn't we all?

Your Turn

Key points, or ... If you don't remember anything else from this chapter, remember this:

- Keep your mind open to therapies that might enhance your existing COPD treatment program.

- Always consult your personal physician before starting additional therapy.
- Check credentials and references of anyone who will be coaching you on movement or performing body contact therapy.

Ask yourself this:

- Could yoga, tai chi, or massage help me?

This week:

- Ask a respiratory health care professional or a peer with COPD if they would recommend this type of therapy.

Here's more help

- *The Healing Massage: A Practical Guide to Relaxation and Well-Being,* by Susan Mumford

Losing Someone with COPD
[JVT/JMM]

Life is a great sunrise. I do not see why
death should not be an even greater one.
– Vladimir Nobokov

Life's Lessons
[JVT]

Sadly, we recently lost two of our COPD support group members. They passed away on the same day.

Elizabeth seemed to be such a gentle lady, and was enthusiastic about joining our group and coming to meetings. Jack was just irrepressible – so full of life, and with such a zest for living! Jack, I believe, never met a stranger. He could – and did – converse with anyone who showed the least interest in talking with him. He took up many of the causes that were offered specifically for supplemental oxygen users, and came away with numerous friends each time. He just had a special delight in his eyes... mischievous, yes, harmful to others, never!

Losing Jack has made me think about the valiant fight he put forth as he battled COPD. In recent months his health took a nosedive, and he struggled mightily to regain his strength and stamina. He never did.

But more than that, Jack's life was open and loving, and accepting, and totally nonjudgmental. We can all learn from that. And we can all strive to embrace the positive aspects of our lives, now. Even with COPD. Just as Jack did.

Okay, I know it's no fun living with obstructive lung disease. But we still have our vision, which allows us to see the beautiful things – and people – around us. We still have our hearts, and although they may be a little rusty from the strain of pumping against impaired lung function, these organs allow us feelings of love and affection, or so the fable of the heart goes.

At least some of us still have our hearing, which brings us the joy of pleasant sounds and wonderful music, of soft voices and babies' excited laughter. We still have our brains, mostly intact, which let us remember the good times and the great people we've known, some who came directly from our involvement with our breathing support group. We can listen when friends and family talk to us, and really hear the meaning behind the words.

We still have a lot to be thankful for, and with many more good things to come. Sometimes it takes the loss of a friend to make us realize that, in spite of COPD, we can have a really good life.

We can still laugh, and yes, sometimes we cry. We may not be able to run anymore, but we can walk. Most of all, we must remember that we should never, ever take for granted the life we live.

Take a page from Jack's book. Live your life with joy in your heart, and don't be afraid to share it with others.

Losing Friends in Pulmonary Rehab
[JMM]

In memory of "The Three Amigos," Arnie, Les and Merle.

Probably the hardest aspect of my job as a respiratory therapist in pulmonary rehab is losing a patient, to death. Often, the participants in our program become friends, the class members become like family. Cohesive. Bonded. The group, as well as our staff, can't help but be affected when a member passes away.

So, what to do? How to cope when you know you all have the same, or similar, incurable, progressive disease? Even if the person who died didn't pass away as a direct result of his or her pulmonary disease, their passing reminds us of our own mortality. Sometimes classmates will wonder aloud, "Am I next?"

As we process the loss, we as a pulmonary rehab program have our own special ways to grieve, remember, and honor the memory of our classmates. I hope you have your own things you do, as well, that hold meaning for you.

Below are some things we do, call them customs, call them rituals. We call them honoring our friends. We call them comforting.

We post a picture of the departed classmate along with his or her obituary in the sign-in area. This way, participants are informed at the beginning of class what has happened. They then have at minimum an hour together to share memories, or at the very least, not be alone.

A dear lady in one class brings in a long-stemmed cut flower and places it on the chair where that person sat.

We all, classmates and staff, sign a sympathy card to send to the family.

If possible, some staff and classmates individually attend the wake, visitation, or funeral. It means so much to the family to meet people who knew their loved one. Even though some have never met the people from pulmonary rehab, the person's family members feel they know us because they've heard their loved one often talk about us at home, about us. If we can't attend services or visitation, we may make a short phone call to a family member.

Some participants in our program have learned how to raise monarch butterflies. There's a tradition in my family, and now with those in our pulmonary rehab program, to name a Monarch when it is released – to give it the name of someone lost within the past year. Seeing a brand new butterfly spread its wings and fly, while calling it by the name of your lost loved one is a healing experience, and an affirmation that life is eternal.

When we lose a friend in pulmonary rehab, yes, our grief is great. But if we wish, as a class, a group, peers, students, friends, we can feel free to share our grief, our joy, even tears. It doesn't make it any easier, but it does give us comfort.

Maybe the classmate lost was quiet and reserved. Maybe he or she was the class clown or perhaps the nurturer, the den mother (or father). No matter what, we are thankful for the way in which they contributed to our group. We honor them by being thankful in this way, thankful that they were a part of our experience, our journey to better health. But perhaps the greatest honor we can bestow is simply to never forget them.

Do Not Stand at My Grave and Weep

Do not stand at my grave and weep,
I am not there, I do not sleep.
I am in a thousand winds that blow,
I am the softly falling snow.
I am the gentle showers of rain,
I am the fields of ripening grain.
I am in the morning hush,
I am in the graceful rush
Of beautiful birds in circling flight,
I am the starshine of the night.
I am in the flowers that bloom,

I am in a quiet room.
I am in the birds that sing,
I am in each lovely thing.
Do not stand at my grave and cry,
I am not there.
I do not die.

– Mary Elizabeth Frye*

(*Reprinted around the world as "Anonymous" for many years, this moving poem was most recently attributed to Mary Elizabeth Frye, written in 1937, and verified by the research of newspaper columnist, Abigail Van Buren in 1998; although some ambiguity remains.)

Your Turn

Key points, or . . . If you don't remember anything else from this chapter, remember this:

- It's a fact of life that at some time or another we will lose friends and loved ones who have the same, or similar health issue.
- Spending time with others who knew that person is helpful, even if in silence.
- Participating in customs or rituals is comforting and helps us heal, even though we're still sad.

Ask yourself this:

- Do I express appreciation, even if it's just a smile or friendly hello to those I know who have serious health problems?

This week:

- Take special notice of the positive qualities in those you know and love, and tell those folks that you appreciate them.

Here's more help

- *Healing After Loss: Daily Meditations For Working Through Grief,* by Martha Whitmore Hickman.
- *Why Me? Coping With Grief, Loss and Change,* by Pesach Krauss.

Isolation with COPD and Why We Need Emotional Support

[JVT]

Individually, we are one drop. Together, we are an ocean.
– Ryunosuke Satoro

Someone in the medical profession once said to me, "People with COPD are like old Indians – they tend to just fade away." What that person was referring to was the fact that many of us have a tendency disappear from the public eye, to stay at home where it is easier and more comfortable than venturing out. COPD itself isn't to blame for the isolation. We aren't contagious. But there are many considerations that lead to our decision to "stay in."

A serious lack of energy is one of the reasons we tend to stay at home. Getting ready to be seen by the outside world requires a great deal of effort. We have to shower, maybe shampoo, shave or apply makeup, and dress. These are not small tasks when each one may send us grasping for our puffers and gasping for breath.

Then there is the issue of embarrassment. We may be embarrassed when we're out in public because of sensitivity about our oxygen equipment or because we may be seized with a spell of uncontrollable coughing. We might feel uncomfortable because we can only walk for short distances before exhaustion sets in, or perhaps because people stare at us. Maybe we simply don't feel well. It's hard to get out and about on those bad days. All of these are reasons we can become mired in isolation.

Isolation is a killer for COPD patients. It may take us away far sooner than even a series of exacerbations. It is something we need to fight with all the energy we can muster, because the alternative is simply to give in to seclusion – and cause us just to fade away!

Granted, it takes a lot of effort for us to socialize. And no one around us will ever understand the price we pay to go to a movie or have lunch with friends. It will never occur to them the kind of effort it takes for us to get out to enjoy a birthday party. Nor should it. We have to realize that we are the ones who must be aware of the importance of getting on with our lives, and to do it with all the quality we can hold on to. We should not depend on others – even caregivers or mates – to provide us with entertainment and a reason to live.

As people with COPD, we don't have to be isolated. By being realistic about our abilities as well as our limitations, we can implement a plan that will provide us with plenty of reasons to get up each day.

Below is a list of relatively easy-to-do activities, even for COPDers.

* Make a list of people you enjoy being with – people who are good for you – people who have a positive attitude. Plan some activities or events that will allow you to spend time with them. Refer to your list often, and remind yourself why you need to be with them.
* Plan your calendar, keeping in mind the activities that take the most effort. Space your outings so there is plenty of rest time in between.

* Keep things simple! If you are inviting folks over for lunch, plan a menu that will be easy, not one that requires huge amounts of effort. Choose a salad that can be prepared the day before. Select a dessert you can pick up from the local bakery. It's the company that counts, not the praise for being a great host.

Make a list of things you really like to do. Is it reading, playing bridge, attending craft fairs, playing with your grandchildren, baking, solving puzzles, updating a scrapbook or family photo album, corresponding with faraway friends? How about going to the movies, lunch or dinner out, attending church or your synagogue, or taking a scenic drive? These are things you can plan to enjoy with someone, breaking the isolation. The important thing is to do them! Don't just plan. Carry them out!

We can't forget how much it helps to go to support group meetings. Involvement in a COPD Support Group is a good place to start breaking a habit of isolation. The people we meet there share many of the same symptoms, concerns, and issues. It really does help to go to meetings – to listen, to talk, to learn, to exchange experiences, and to share feelings with those who truly understand how we feel.

Pulmonary rehab is another great way to get out and meet people who understand what we're going through. Even if we don't feel like going anywhere, if we're not sick that day, we should push ourselves to get there. After we do, we're so glad we did!

Finally, avoiding isolation and getting out is a commitment to ourselves that we are going to work to feel better, or at least remain stable. It's a commitment we should be happy to make, for the results of our involvement far outweigh our effort. We'll feel so much better because of the company, the activity, the experience. Our hearts will be lighter, and so will the burden of our disease.

Living with COPD is not a death sentence. It's a journey. And when we're walking a path we've never been on before, it sure does help to have some friends with a map.

Your Turn

Key points, or . . . If you don't remember anything else from this chapter, remember this:

- No matter what level of COPD you have, you must avoid isolation as much as possible.
- You can still have a social life, even if you are significantly limited by your COPD.
- Becoming involved in a breathing support group and / or pulmonary rehab is a good place to start and a way to meet others.

Ask yourself this:

- Do I regularly get out in public and socialize with others? If so, what do I do? If not, why not?

This week:

- Do at least one of the following:
- Find your nearest breathing support group and make plans to attend.
- Find your nearest Pulmonary Rehabilitation Program, talk with the staff and ask if it would be appropriate for you to enroll.
- Call a friend or family member and set a date to do something you enjoy.

Here's more help

- The American Lung Association has a listing of breathing support groups throughout the United States. Visit them online at http://www.lungusa. org, call 800 LUNG-USA (800-598-8252), or call your local hospital to ask about a group near you.
- The American Association for Cardiovascular and Pulmonary Rehabilitation (AACVPR) has a listing of pulmonary rehab programs throughout the United States and beyond. Visit them online at http://www.aacvpr.org, call them at 312-321-5146, email: aacvpr@aacvpr.org, or call your local hospital to ask about a group near you.

Ten Tips for Enjoying the Holidays
[JMM]

*Don't let what you cannot do interfere
with what you can do.*
– John Wooden

If you're healthy and free of chronic disease, the holidays can be stressful enough. But, if you have COPD you might be looking at the holidays with downright fear and trepidation, and be inclined to say, "It's such a hassle. I'm tempted to forget the whole thing and just stay home." Trust me. It doesn't have to be that way!

Here are ten tips to help you enjoy the holidays, even if you have COPD. This is, by no means, a complete list – it's just a start to show you that with a little planning – and some clever thinking – you can get out, participate in holiday events and enjoy the season with family and friends.

1. **Scented candles** – If you're going to a party or gathering where you expect there might be scented candles, call ahead and gently ask your host if they would mind not lighting them that day, or at least until after you've left the party. Explain that the scent irritates your lungs and you won't be able to appreciate the party if the candles get in the way of your ability to breathe.

2. **Park close or be dropped off** – Don't find yourself walking farther than you're comfortably able to walk, especially in the cold air. If you're riding

with someone, ask if they can drop you off at the door. If you're doing the driving, call ahead to your host and ask if you can drive up to the door and someone at the party (perhaps a responsible teen driver) can serve as a valet. This is where having a cell phone comes in handy. Everyone with COPD should have a cell phone when they venture away from home!

3. **Don't eat too much** – All those goodies are tempting, but overeating can expand your stomach to the point that it pushes up on your already compromised diaphragm. Want to try everything? You can. Don't gobble it all down at once; just take little bits and bites, and stretch it out over time.

4. **Give yourself time** – Rushing and hurrying is a huge problem for people with breathing problems who simply can't move fast. Allow for plenty of time to get ready so you'll arrive when you want, look beautiful / handsome (whatever the case may be) and have breath to spare!

5. **Avoid nasty germs** – Stay away from small children who are coughing and sneezing. At their age they don't know enough to cover their mouth and nose. As uppity as it may sound, avoid shaking hands and kissing on the lips. Most people can shake off a cold virus. You can't! The Hollywood "air kiss" works just fine. When you've weathered the winter without an exacerbation, you'll be happy you did – or didn't!

6. **Cover up** – Wear a mask or scarf over your nose and mouth in cold air to keep your airways from having spasms, which causes an uncontrollable cough and more shortness of breath.

7. **Delegate** – Shop for gifts online. If you can't, ask someone to go shopping with you or to pick up a specific, easy-to-find gift when they're out doing their shopping. If the party's at your house, don't do all the work! Involve your guests and assign tasks. Children, and yes, even teens, are usually willing to help – and be shown some appreciation for doing so. It will enrich their lives to learn about your physical limitations and it will make them feel proud to know they've helped out.

8. **Be a Santa** – Surprise someone by doing something nice. Send a note to your neighbor or phone a friend with a brief and cheerful, "I'm just thinking about you and wanted to wish you a "Merry Christmas" or "Happy Hanukkah." Make cookies or a quick bread for your letter carrier. Never underestimate the power of a small, but kind, deed. Little things really do mean a lot!

9. **Enjoy the moments** – Live in the moment. If you're breathing well at the moment, smile, laugh, and enjoy the party! Don't spend your energy worrying about tomorrow. This very day – the time you're in right now – will never come along again. All of us are promised only today, nothing else.

10. **It's their problem** – Don't beat yourself up over what you might have done in the past to cause damage to your lungs. You're not the only person at that party who may have done something bad for their health. You're doing the very best you can right now to be healthy, and if someone can't deal with that, it's their problem. If you use supplemental oxygen (and we say supplemental because *everybody* uses oxygen) think of it this way: Some people use bottled water, you just used bottled air!

Your Turn

Key points, or... If you don't remember anything else from this chapter, remember this:

- Plan ahead.
- Know your limits.
- Cherish the moment.
- Have fun!

Ask yourself this:

- What was a problem for me last year? Can any of these suggestions help make my holidays more enjoyable this year?

This week:

- Think about an upcoming event and make arrangements to make it enjoyable for you.

Here's more help

- COPD-International –Conserving Energy: http://www.copd-international.com/Library/living-series-energy.htm
- See Chapter December – Week 2 – Party Time! Nine Ways to Help You Save Energy and Breathe Better this Holiday Season

A Time of Thanksgiving
[JVT]

Not what we say about our blessings, but how we
use them, is the true measure of our thanksgiving.
– W.T.Purkiser

In the United States we honor a tradition with our observance of Thanksgiving Day, a day of family and feasting, and of expressing our thanks for all we have.

It seems to me that those of us with COPD may have our own special reasons to celebrate and give thanks. Our perspective, coming from that of having been diagnosed with a chronic, progressive, so-far-incurable disease, may be different and more specific than others in our world, because it comes from the unique mind set of someone who must struggle each day to breathe well, to survive to see tomorrow.

Let's count our blessings together. Some of yours may be different than mine, but I know that we share many of the same reasons to give thanks. I picture a cornucopia not with what I don't have, but what I do. This is what I see:

* I am grateful to have the strength it takes to get up and face each new day.
* I give thanks for each time I am able to avoid a lung infection.
* I am more appreciative than ever of the beauty that surrounds me – in nature, in my life, in my heart.
* I am thankful for the support and understanding of my family and good friends.

* I am glad I have more good days than bad ones.
* I am pleased I can rely on my doctor and health-care team in times of need.
* I am grateful for the friends I have made in our support group – people who truly understand how I feel.
* I am deliriously happy with the extra mobility that my portable oxygen system provides, and with all of the innovations in supplemental oxygen delivery systems.
* I am delighted to know that research is taking place that may provide insight and help for all COPDers.
* I am grateful for the pleasure I derive from short walks by the ocean.
* I am happy I can occasionally dream that I am healthy again, freed in my dreams from the disability of COPD.
* If you are lucky enough to have a spouse who watches over you and helps you, you are glad to be able to say "Thank You!" to him or her.

Thanksgiving does not have to be marked on a calendar. It can be honored each day. It doesn't need to be accompanied by roast turkey and all the trimmings. It can be a quiet, solitary meal, or a simple acknowledgement of the importance of those individuals who affect our lives so deeply now. You know who they are, and so should they.

As pulmonary patients, our perspectives may be different, but our passions are as strongly felt as anyone else's. And I suspect that the gratitude we feel for the continuance of the good things in our lives may be even more heartfelt because we are constantly at risk of losing them.

Each of us occasionally gives in to brief bouts of grieving for the things that we can no longer do or have. However, as the changes in our lifestyles have taken place, so, too, have new opportunities found their way to us. Those new doors that have been opened are the ones we must focus on now. They are the promise of good times to come, of cherished memories – and new beginnings.

Those newly discovered opportunities are huge reasons, themselves, for our gratitude. *Anticipation, excitement, joy, and a sense of accomplishment* – all are by-products of taking on new responsibilities and learning about new pleasures. All can bring renewal and rediscovery to each of us. I am so grateful to be aware of them in my life.

When I face each day as a precious gift, I feel grateful. The gift of a new day is the best one we can expect to receive. Think about it – with the dawn of each new day it's like getting God's okay to have another go at it. So, let's take it, do our best, and just say, "Thank you."

Your Turn

Key points, or … If you don't remember anything else from this chapter, remember this:

- It's not just good, but good for us to be thankful for whatever we have.
- We can find many things to be thankful for if we just take the time to notice them.
- Having COPD may take some things away but it can also give us new opportunities.

Ask yourself this:

- Because I have COPD, what good things are in my life now that I didn't have before?

This week:

- Find something to be thankful for each day this week and write it down on this page or you can somewhere else, but just write it down. At the end of the week look back on it.

Sunday – I am thankful for _____

_____

Monday – I am thankful for _____

_____

Tuesday – I am thankful for _____

_____

Wednesday – I am thankful for _____

_____

Thursday – I am thankful for _____

_____

Friday – I am thankful for_____

_____

Saturday – I am thankful for_____

_____

Here's more help

- Breathing Better Living Well thankfulness forum. http://www.breathingbetterlivingwell.com/community.php
- *Thank You Power,* by Deborah Norville.
- *Choosing Gratitude: Your Journey to Joy,* by Nancy Leigh DeMoss

Excerpted from "A Time of Thanksgiving" written by Jane M. Martin, BA, LRT, CRT and published on COPDConnection.com. Copyright 2010 HealthCentral. All rights reserved. http://www.healthcentral.com/copd/c/19257/124748/time-thanksgiving/?ic=4027

Dear Family and Friends
In a Perfect World...
[JVT]

Learn what you are, and be such.
– Pindar

Dear Family and Friends,

In a perfect world, I wouldn't have COPD. Yet, I do, and because of that, our lives may never be quite the same, A.D. (after diagnosis). But we can all try to seek more joy, derive more pleasure, from what we are fortunate enough to have – one another. Let's make the most of our time.

In a perfect world, you wouldn't have to wonder how I was feeling, and wonder what you might be able to do to help me. You wouldn't find yourself on the receiving end of my reactions to the depression spells to which I am prone. Nor would you have to puzzle over the fact that I seem to have good days, and then unexplainably, so many bad days.

You must be terribly disturbed by my shortness of breath, and by the fatigue that nibbles at me all day, every day. And I can guess that you are as upset and embarrassed as I am by the fits of coughing that sometimes seize me, especially out in public.

You know that the compromises to my lifestyle are upsetting. It's hard for me to ask for help when I find that I can no longer do something on my own. It hurts my pride, and I can see in your eyes that it hurts you, too.

But it isn't a perfect world, is it? I do have this disease, and so far there is no cure for it. I must learn to cope with it. We all must. So, even though my world is less than perfect, particularly since being diagnosed with COPD, these issues do exist. I want to find a way to help you as you try to help me. That's why I'm writing this letter to you now. Sometimes it's just easier to write things down than it is to say them out loud – especially things that cause this big lump in my throat, even as I write.

You are my loved and cherished family. And it seems to me that family members are often hit as hard with the realities of COPD as the patient. Maybe even harder. It pains me to see you struggle with solutions as we fight the battle of this disease together. I know you want to help.

Our lives cannot help but be affected by the fact that I have this disease. But I have learned that COPD is not a death sentence, nor does it have to be the end of our quality of life. The better I become at managing my own disease, the more effective and happier our time together will be. Maybe if we establish some ground rules, we can get through the rough patches and adapt more easily and with less stress on us all.

Here is my fantasy of what our nearly perfect world could be – in spite of COPD – within my list of seven suggestions:

1. It is important for me to remain as independent as possible to preserve my self-esteem. Try not to rush to help me before you know whether or not I can accomplish a task on my own. I really want to try; not only to spare you, but also to help me with my independence and self esteem, both of which will erode significantly with everything I learn I can't do.

There is a fine line that you, my dear ones, must walk in balancing between coming to my aid, or just taking over for me (which can be interpreted as enabling me to become a cripple). This is important for many reasons: The need to keep my body and muscles as conditioned and toned as possible, and the need I have to feel useful again – to help guard against a loss of self esteem.

2. Try to not judge me if I'm having a bad day. It is possible that a lung infection could be brewing, and you may be aware of it sooner than I am myself. You know the signs... increased shortness of breath and coughing up discolored sputum. Perhaps fever, but maybe not, and less energy to expend on the simple chores of daily living.

   Some of the folks in my lung support group have expressed their frustration when their family leaps to the conclusion that we are hypochondriacs who complain a lot about feeling bad. This just isn't so; we aren't constant complainers. COPDers are a pretty brave lot. Our malady may not be visible, but it is real.

   Most of us who have COPD do not want our loved ones to see us as "sickly" or making excuses. As a result, however, many of us hedge about the problems we are having.

3. Please help me by overseeing that I am complying with my doctor's treatment plan. I don't expect you to be a nurse, but I appreciate it if you gently remind me to take my afternoon puffs on my inhalers, or to confirm that I remembered to take my evening pills. Help me be a compliant patient by assisting with my oxygen equipment

when we go out. It's good to know I have a portable filled with enough supplemental oxygen to get me comfortably through our schedule.

It's also good to have help getting in and out of the car, and especially supportive to have an arm to lean on going up stairs, if I need it. The more comfortable we all are with the oxygen and equipment, the sooner it will be accepted and not questioned by the general public.

4. Help me stay socialized. Do not let me become isolated from friends and other family members. We COPD folks do have a tendency to stay at home rather than digging down deep for the energy to get up and out! You can encourage me to go with you to lunch, or even to the market. You can inspire me to go to a movie or to have guests in for bridge, scrabble or cribbage. Your encouragement makes the difference for me – desiring to see people, and for people to see me!

5. In this nearly perfect world, we need to have and show respect for one another. I promise I won't talk about you as if you aren't in the room, if you'll do the same for me. My feelings are worn very close to the surface; I can hear perfectly well what you've said to someone about how fast the disease is progressing, or about how futile our efforts to fight it may seem. You and I can certainly discuss these issues between ourselves, and keep them within the family circle.

6. Encourage me (but please don't nag me) about getting my exercises in each day. Some days it is just so hard to commit to even ten minutes of active exercises. If I'm too sick to do them myself, try to help me with just some stretching exercises

like yoga or tai chi. These gentle movements can help to keep my body conditioned, even when I'm suffering from an exacerbation. And they aren't that taxing of my strength or energy. You, of course, no matter how hard you try, cannot fully understand how I am feeling because you don't have COPD. But your encouragement brings me added strength; your emotional support brings me peace from the trauma of being sick.

7. Nutrition is an important part of helping my body with its special needs. You can help by making sure I'm eating right. A diet high in protein will help build up my immune system and body strength. We can plan the week's menus together. I pledge to try and tell you what items seem to taste best to me.

That's it. I'll stop with Lucky #7. I don't wish to make our lives more difficult with suggestions and rules. I simply want to express myself on the subject of how you can help me. I don't want to sound as though I am whining or complaining. I am reaching out with all the love in my heart for the help I know you want to provide. And if you have your own list of suggestions, please share them with me.

It is true that our lives may never be quite the same. But we can work together to preserve and enhance what we are fortunate enough to have – one another. Help me continue to fight, to become stable, to endure what I will not let bring me down. Let's make the most of our time.

From my heart to yours,

Your Person with COPD

Your Turn

Key points, or . . . If you don't remember anything else from this chapter, remember this:

- Your family members want to help you in the best way possible. Sometimes they just don't know how.
- Open communication with your family and friends will help you all to understand how to cope with COPD.

Ask yourself this:

- Have I told my loved ones what I need from them and what I don't need?

This week:

- If this letter explains the way you feel, show it to your family and / or friends. If you feel differently, think about writing your own letter.

Here's more help

- Love Your Lungs Breathe for Life – Information and support for families of people with COPD; http:// www.loveyourlungsbreatheforlife.com
- Well Spouse Foundation (for family members and other caregivers) – 800-838-0879, http:// www.wellspouse.org

War or Peace?

[JVT/JMM]

*Acceptance doesn't mean you're giving up, or giving in.
It means, simply, that you're smart enough to know
what's going on so you can do what you need to do
to live your life as well as you can.*
– Iris Carlyle

No matter what your spiritual belief, the holiday season should be a time of peace and well-being. The ideal would be to have peace with our family, our friends, our fellow man. But is it possible to make peace with a raging chronic disease that at times seems to spiral out of control, beyond our reach, with as little as a cough or sneeze? And how do we have peace within if some choices we make now or have made in the past aggravate or have lead in part to the development of COPD?

Have you ever noticed that some people seem to cope, emotionally, with COPD much better than others? Why is that? Possibly because they've found a way to stop being angry with themselves; they've made their way past the rage that often comes as a part of living with COPD.

Perhaps they have learned, also, to avoid – or at least work through – the occasional bouts of depression that commonly come with COPD. They have accepted the role of exercise as a vital part of their routine and most of them follow the treatment plan of their pulmonary doctor, actively involved in the management of their COPD.

They are educated about the disease. They are knowledgeable about their boundaries – when to push them, when to conserve precious energy and how to make choices that will preserve their quality of life, even with the physical restrictions with which they are presented.

What about smoking? Those of us who were smokers, or still may be, often have an ongoing struggle with quitting – or remaining smoke-free. It can help to avoid fighting mode by simply accepting the fact that we were smokers and always will be. We are those who take one day at a time with the goal to not smoke today.

It's not easy to make peace with COPD. It's a constant presence in the lives of us who live with it. It has a profound impact on our emotional health, self-image, relationships, work habits, aspirations, and overall outlook on life. And our struggle with it can cause us to feel like we've lost control of not only our breathing, but our lives.

It's interesting that the language of disease is a language of combat: We battle cancer, fight infections, overcome paralysis, conquer our fears. Disease is an enemy to be fought, and chronic disease is an enemy that is ever present, threatening us with chaos at any time. The war imagery obligates us to resist. On the other hand, looking at ourselves as "victims" of disease indicates that we are passive, when, in fact, chronic disease demands an active response.

What should we do? Should we fight the illness to the death, or live in constant fear of being at the mercy of the next cough or sneeze? As COPD patients, we are neither perfectly healthy nor hopelessly ill. Choice is our right – but balance should be our goal.

Below is a list of scenarios, each with two extreme choices, and a broad spectrum of responses. Neither of these extremes is healthy and they, each in their own way, put us at war with COPD. Where are you?

* You can tough it out, ignoring symptoms at the risk of getting worse – or you can check out every little quirk, at the risk of hypochondria.
* You can shop for miracle cures at the risk of harming yourself – or you can blindly trust one doctor's judgment at the risk of selecting unwisely.
* You can keep your disease secret at the risk of deception – or you can talk about it often at the risk of self-pity.
* You can hold fast to your independence at the risk of isolation and pushing yourself – or you can constantly ask friends for help at the risk of becoming a burden.
* You can insist that your family treat you as normal and healthy at the risk of denying them the right to be concerned about you – or you can let them coddle you at the risk of becoming dependent and childlike.
* You can strain your body to its limits at the risk of harming yourself – or you can play it too safe at the risk of becoming an invalid.
* You can look upon each good day as if you've "beaten the system" at the risk of smugness – or you can live in terror of degeneration and death at the risk of being emotionally paralyzed.
* You can insist on controlling every single aspect of your life at the risk of frustration – or you can "go with the flow" at the risk of passivity and victimization.
* You can be angry about your fate at the risk of bitterness – or you can focus only on your blessings at the risk of self-delusion.

War or Peace? The choices we make each day determine how we live with COPD. It isn't easy, but we can live in peace with COPD by having the grace of acceptance, and the determination to seek improvement. No doubt there will be days in which we won't make the right choices, but we'll learn from our mistakes. And we will keep on trying and also learn from others. With good choices, we'll have the peace that comes with doing the best we can under all circumstances. Our own balanced and centered life will get us through the rough times, and will define who we are, with or without COPD.

Bonus Box
Shame and Guilt with Smoking – or –
"What do I Expect? I Had It Coming."
[JMM]

Not all COPD is caused by cigarette smoking[5], but let's face it – most of it, about 85%, is. If you smoked cigarettes (or are still a smoker) and have COPD, you may be feeling guilty or ashamed for "bringing this on yourself."

So, how do you make peace with the thought of having an incurable, progressive illness that could have been prevented? First, know you're not the only person who ever smoked and got COPD. There are millions like you. Next, know that you can find support from those who have been there, support in quit smoking classes and breathing support groups.

The people there are ready to help you. your doctor about recommending a quit method that may work for you. Choose a quit date that's meaningful *to you*

5. Secondhand smoke, air pollution, chemical fumes, dust from the environment or workplace, and genetically inherited Alpha-1 Antitrypsin Deficiency can contribute to COPD. Source: National Heart, Lung and Blood Institute. 2010.

and / or a loved one: A birthday, anniversary, graduation, etc., with hopes do, just start. Take one step at a time, and if you fall down, just get up and keep on trying.

Not all COPD is caused by cigarette smoking, but let's face it – most of it, about 85%, is. If you smoked cigarettes (or are still a smoker) and have COPD, you may be feeling guilty or ashamed for "bringing this on yourself."

So, how do you make peace with the thought of having an incurable, progressive illness that could have been prevented? First, know you're not the only person who ever smoked and got COPD. There are millions like you. Next, know that you can find support from those who have been there, support in quit smoking classes and breathing support groups. The people there are ready to help you.

Ask your doctor about recommending a quit method that may work for you. Choose a quit date that's meaningful to you and / or a loved one: A birthday, anniversary, graduation, etc., with hopes for celebrating many more to come! Whatever you do, just start. Take one step at a time, and if you fall down, just get up and keep on trying.

Below are some letters of support from folks who were past smokers, and heavily addicted to nicotine. They did it. I hope you can, too.

Dear Betty,
I can relate. I was afraid to give up cigarettes as they were my best friends. I thought an hour without one seemed impossible, so I began by doing without one for only five minutes at a time. I had a desire to smoke, but it went away whether I smoked or not. That's how I got through it. If it were easy, everyone would quit. It was the hardest thing I ever did, but that keeps some of the guilt

in check. Remember, you will go though many emotions and should feel free to express them. Don't keep your fears to yourself. Good luck.

   Linda

Hi Kay!

   Just wanted to let you know that the craving does lessen. The more time that goes by, the less the urge. For me, it was hard to get past that hand-mouth thing. So, I stuffed my mouth with hard candy and food, not the best way . . . just substituting one addiction for another. Before I quit I didn't know that the car would start without a cigarette, or that I could talk on the phone without one. Tea, alone? Without a butt? Impossible! But that passed. For a long time after I quit, I had the smoking dream . . . the one where I would light up and wake up in a panic, breaking out into a cold sweat. It was before my COPD diagnosis, during my long denial period, and yet, even then, I knew that one more butt would kill me because there was no such thing as only 'one.'

   Today, I rarely get the urge except after I put the Thanksgiving turkey in the oven. In years past, that was the time I would sit for a few minutes, feet up, and light up . . . a short break before beginning the rest of the cooking. For the last three years, we've gone to a dear friend for that holiday. No more urges for that day!

   Seriously, it really does pass. It's just hard to see when recovery is so new. Just take it one day at a time – it's the only way to survive it! Seriously, it really does pass. It's just hard to see when recovery is so new. Just take it one day at a time – it's the only way to survive it!

Arlene
I quit smoking three times before the success would last. The first time I threw my cigarettes out the car window. I just threw them out. And I went through all the cravings for about six months. The second time I took a Smoke Stoppers class through work. The third time, I went out and bought a pound of candy – you know, all the mixed candies you buy in bulk. Every time I craved a cigarette, I'd have a piece of candy. I never really liked sweets. About half way through the second pound, I just quit. That was it. I quit for good.
John

Finally, here is a letter to all the new quitters in a COPD online support group. The cheerleader is Janie in Sacramento, California.

Hello Everyone,
It's been a week now since you had that last cigarette. And this isn't the letter that I had prepared for the first anniversary week for new non-smokers. The original was pretty typical jargon, you know, the 'atta girl' and 'atta boy' routine.
Then yesterday I heard the results of a Pulmonary Function test from one of my best friends who recently celebrated her 60th bithday. Due primarily to not being able to stop smoking, her lung function had dropped 10% in the past two and a half years. She had felt so guilty about smoking that she canceled checkups with her pulmonary doctor until she stopped three months ago. It made me wonder how highly intelligent men and

women could fall prey to a tobacco leaf that only an insect would eat. It made me wonder how easy it is for us to say, 'I'll think about that tomorrow' or 'I'll stop as a New Year's resolution next year.' It made me wonder why we ignored the warning signs. It made me wonder about a lot of things we would rather not confront.

For all of you out there who are 'hanging in there,' you should be very proud of what you are doing for yourselves and for your families. If you temporarily fail, dust yourself off and get back up again. But don't stop trying!

Playing solitaire in your bathrobe 24 / 7 is better than O$_2$ 24 / 7. Eating carrot sticks, lemon drops, jellybeans, or carrying water everywhere is better than having a cigarette. I once knew a CEO who ate toothpicks after he gave up smoking. He nibbled them and then spit out the little pieces of wood during board meetings. Disgusting to eat wood? And okay to ingest tobacco smoke? Well, you decide.

Just don't give up! We are cheering for all of you . . . those of you who were brave enough to come out and admit to everyone that you were trying to quit, and those of you who are quietly trying to stop in your own way. We are here to help you find a better life than tobacco can give you. We're listening!

Janie in Sacramento

Your Turn

Key points, or ... If you don't remember anything else from this chapter, remember this:

- It is normal, and human, to feel as if you're at war with your COPD.

- You can learn how to make good choices – and keep a balance – for control of your disease, and your life.

Ask yourself this:

- Where am I on the spectrum of responses to life with my chronic pulmonary disease?

This week:

- Do your best to avoid extremes, but have balance in the choices you make to live in peace with lung disease.

Here's more help

- Health Central Smoking Cessation Management http://www.healthcentral.com/copd/manage. html
- *Breathwish: a Scriptural Guide to Smoking Cessation and Understanding COPD*, by Craig Ammerall, RRT.

Party Time! Nine Ways to Help You Save Energy and Breathe Better this Holiday Season

[JMM]

> *Nothing is particularly hard if*
> *you divide it into small jobs.*
> – Henry Ford

The holidays are upon us, and if you're anything like me, you're wondering how you're going to fit everything in and still have time to enjoy this merry season. If you're living with COPD, especially, taking part in all this activity might seem like way too much to tackle. You might be thinking, "I barely have enough energy and enough breath, as it is. How am I going to survive – let alone enjoy – the holidays?"

Below are some tips to help you conserve that precious energy – and breath – so you can take pleasure in a joyful holiday season. In the November – Week 2 chapter we talked about some general holiday issues to consider. Here we're going to talk specifically about **saving your energy** to make holiday tasks easier.

1. **Prioritize** – Which events do you really want to attend, and which ones are actually more an obligation to make someone else happy? Do what means the most to *you* and politely tell

your friends and loved ones that you have only so much breath to go around. Maybe you can do something fun with them after the first of the year when life is not so hectic.

2. **Position yourself** – If you're at a family gathering and you want to help but don't have a lot of energy or endurance, ask if there is something you can do while sitting down. Maybe you can arrange a veggie or deli platter, fold napkins, or wrap gifts. If you have trouble standing for an extended period of time, don't volunteer to do the dishes. Rather, you might sit at the table and dry them. Guys, this goes for you, too!

3. **Plan ahead** – Being in a hurry is one of biggest breath-robbers for people with COPD! Give yourself plenty of time to get ready, gather your goodies, and arrive at your destination with breath to spare.

4. **Place yourself** – Don't seat yourself near triggers such as cooking fumes, steamy pots, scented candles, or stuffy, overly warm areas. Sit where there is more likely to be moving air, near a fan or a cracked-open door or window.

5. **Pack it and pull it** – If you have gifts or other items to bring along, tote them in a rolling cart. If you don't have a cart, leave your packages and potluck dish in the car and ask a more able family member to unload them for you. If neither of these is an option, pack your stuff into a backpack or a tote bag, preferably with a long enough strap to go over your head and across your chest. It helps to carry a load close to the core of your body rather than in your hands. This also can

keep your hands free to hold on to a railing or the arm of a friend.

6. **Push it** – Use a grocery cart every time you shop, even if you're not buying a lot. Wipe the handle with an anti-bacterial towelette before you grab it. Ask the bagger to pack your bags light. More, lightweight bags are easier to carry than a few heavy ones.

7. **Pump it up** – Although it might be tempting to skip pulmonary rehab class or routine exercise over the holidays, keep in mind that exercise helps reduce stress and also burns off the extra calories you're likely to consume around this time of year. Besides, it's fun to celebrate the holidays with your friends at pulmonary rehab. If you absolutely don't have the time or energy for aerobic exercise, at least do your stretches and strength training. It will keep you feeling good, and flexible.

8. **Pucker up and Pace** – Use your breathing techniques! You know (or at least I hope you do) that pursed-lips breathing really does make a difference in helping you stay in control of your breathing. Slow down and remind yourself to do it, even if you have to count it out: In one, two...Out one, two, three, four. Ahhhh...

9. **Puff your O$_2$** – If your doctor has prescribed oxygen, wear it. Everybody at that party needs oxygen – for every breath they take. You just happen to need a little more. Give your body a break and nourish it with O$_2$. You will have more energy and your lungs, heart, and brain, will be a lot less stressed!

It's Party Time! Prioritize, Position, Plan, Pace, Pack, Pull, Push, Pump, Pucker, Pace, and Puff. You'll breathe easier and you'll have a great time!

Your Turn

Key points, or…If you don't remember anything else from this chapter, remember this:

- You can participate in holiday events, even if you have COPD.
- The choices you make, even small ones, can mean the difference between having a good time with easy breathing – or a lousy time, struggling for breath.
- You can make good choices – and you must – especially when you are limited by COPD.

Ask yourself this:

- How can I remember to use these tips when I attend my next event or party?

This week:

- There are nine points in this chapter. Take the three that are the biggest problems for you and visualize yourself following the suggestions and breathing better.

Here's more help

- Holidays with COPD – http://www.squidoo.com/managing-COPD#module59171742

- The Complete Guide to Understanding and Living with COPD: From A COPDer's Perspective, by R.D. Martin
- Read or review chapter May – Week 2 – Make the Most of the Breath you Have: Energy Conservation and Work Simplification.

A COPD Christmas

[Jim Phillips]

Twas the night before Christmas, and all through the house
Not a creature was stirring 'cept me and my spouse.
If you're wondering why, let me do some explaining.
We were doing a thing called bronchial draining.

There I was on my slant board, and she on her knees,
Clapping my chest, while I lay there and wheeze.
When all of a sudden, there arose such a clatter
We ran to the window to see what was the matter.

Imagine our surprise to see out in the yard
An old guy bent over and coughing real hard.
He had a white beard and shiny black boots,
A bag full of gifts and wore a red suit.

As we stared, he stood up, and looking at me,
He said in despair, "I have COPD."
"I've wondered each year when I'm out with my pack
If someone would see when I have an attack.

"I fear that I'm just getting older," said he,
"And soon I'll be on Social Security."
"Come in my dear Santa, and you'll soon be elated,
I'll tell you about being rehabilitated.

"Put yourself in the hands of the team,
Pay close attention and you'll be back on the beam.

The things they will teach will bring you success,
Things like breathing and coughing and handling stress.

"You'll exercise right, with treadmill and weights,
What a change will be seen in your physical state!
You'll eat only good things, watching the pounds,
It'll be a lot easier making your rounds.

"So please, Mr. Santa, give rehab a whirl,
Think of your health for the kids of the world."
He said, "Why you're right, sir, the message is clear,
Rehab's the answer. I'll do it this year!"

And laying a finger aside of his nose,
And pursing his lips, up the chimney he rose.
Using diaphragm breathing, he got on his sleigh,
And with a loud "Merry Christmas!" he went on his way.

*("A COPD Christmas" by the late Jim Phillips, reprinted with per-
mission from Kathleen Sullivan of the American Lung Association
of California.)*

Your Turn

**Key points, or . . . If you don't remember anything else
from this chapter, remember this:**

- Sometimes you have to take a break from learning about COPD and just enjoy yourself and
  have fun!

Ask yourself this:

- Am I keeping a sense of humor and fun
  throughout this holiday season?

This week:

- Share this poem, or another fun story or poem, with friends and family.

Thoughts about the Future
[JVT]

The future is called 'perhaps,' which is the only
possible thing to call it. And the important thing
is not to allow that to scare you.
– Tennessee Williams

It's funny, you know…I never really allowed myself to think much about my future after diagnosis. I was, after all, diagnosed with COPD when I was just fifty-two years old. I received the devastating sentence of this incurable, mostly progressive chronic illness, was told I had between two and five years to live, and had to use supplemental oxygen twenty-four hours a day, seven days a week for the rest of my life.

It took me a long time to work my way through the various stages of acceptance, and to adjust to the lifestyle changes required of me. Some of those adjustments kind of snuck up on me when I wasn't looking and somehow became a part of daily living. Others required commitment and dedication of effort, pulling survival instincts from so deep within me that the intensity still comes as a surprise whenever I think about it.

But survive I did! Even with a grim prognosis, I have somehow come through the obstacle course that God set for me, and I now find myself pushing the finish line even further out front.

You see, there is still so much to do! There are sights to be seen, people to help, words to be spoken, and actions to be taken. And try as I might, I can't seem to cram them all into the space of a day – the measure of time we are all given in a twenty-four hour period – a simple day in which to accomplish all that we set before ourselves.

Strangely, I guess that's what has led me to begin planning ahead for the future. And the future I wouldn't allow myself at first, seems to loom ahead of me now like the proverbial carrot before the nose of the donkey. Take just one more step; do just one more thing; and smell the carrot along the way. Mmmmmm!

I am sometimes startled whenever I catch myself thinking about something I want to do a few years down the road. I suddenly find myself making long-term agreements, signing contracts and leases of several years' duration.

I'll admit, there are times when I prefer to give in to this disease, when I awaken in the morning with a raging headache, or when the fatigue pulls me down as though my feet were mired in molasses. But the whiff of that carrot – my future opportunities to do more, be more, help more…serve to push my feet into action and my brain into gear!

Maintaining stability has allowed me to stay in control of COPD and my overall health. Dr. Tom Petty once said that a disease is an impairment of an organ system, its structure or its function; but an illness is the total impact of that impairment on the life of the person. There is a difference. A person can have COPD, a significant disease – without being constantly sick – without being ill.

I accept the fact that having COPD limits me, but it makes my heart soar to know it does not change the person I am. Accepting myself as a person with COPD who can still be healthy and enjoy life has given me the peace and the confidence to be able to consider – and see – a future! Carry on, my friends, into the New Year with this knowledge, confidence, and joy.

Your Turn

Key points, or... If you don't remember anything else from this chapter, remember this:

- COPD is not a death sentence.
- With knowledge, determination, and a positive attitude you can look forward to the future.

Ask yourself this:

- Do I look at COPD as a loss of lung function, but not the loss of the person I am?

This week:

- List three things you are looking forward to in the New Year.

Here's more help

- *Positive Options for Living with COPD: Self-Help and Treatment for Chronic Obstructive Pulmonary Disease,* by Teri Allen
- *Living a Healthy Life with Chronic Conditions: Self Management of Heart Disease, Arthritis, Diabetes, Asthma, Bronchitis, Emphysema and Others,* by Kate Lorig, Halsted Holman MD, David Sobel, MD, Diana Laurent MPH.

May the New Year bring you Joy and Peace, Health, Happiness and Hope

Author Biographies

Jane M. Martin, BA, LRT, CRT

Jane M. Martin is a respiratory therapist and teacher with over thirty years experience in respiratory care. Working in acute care she became frustrated with the "revolving door" – providing emergency and in-patient care to people with lung disease, only to see them return to the hospital not long after with the same problem. Aware that there are over twelve million people with COPD in the US alone, she was disheartened when time after time patients asked her questions such as, "Am I the only one who has this problem? Where can I learn more about my breathing? What's going to happen to me? How can anyone possibly understand how I feel?"

In response, Jane began developing programs for COPD and asthma, focusing on patient education and improved pulmonary health management at home; most notably, Pulmonary Rehabilitation and a Better Breathers' Support group. In her work in pulmonary rehabilitation Jane was inspired by her patients but concerned for others who suffer with little or no information and support. She knew a connection had to be made; a connection between those people who were lonely, angry, and confused with those who had learned to live well in spite of the physical and emotional obstacles encountered in life with chronic lung disease.

In an effort to bring patients together to help each other, Jane wrote *Breathe Better, Live in Wellness: Winning Your Battle Over Shortness of Breath*, a collection of stories of everyday people with extraordinary and inspiring wisdom, humor, and courage. Her focus was on helping readers see how people with lung disease not only survive – but thrive – in spite of a debilitating condition. To further her efforts Jane created BreathingBetterLivingWell.com, a website providing education and support for people with chronic lung disease, featuring a vibrant forum for pulmonary patients to support one another.

Originally from the Chicago area, Jane holds a bachelor's degree in Education and Language Arts from Hope College and a degree in respiratory care from the California College for Health Sciences. She works as a licensed Respiratory Therapist in Pulmonary Rehabilitation, serves as Director of her website, Breathing Better Living Well, writes a bi-weekly article for Health Central's COPD Connection and is a nationally known speaker. Jane's affiliations include membership in the Michigan Society for Respiratory Care and the American Association for Respiratory Care. She serves on the editorial boards of *The COPD Digest* and *Alpha-1 to One*.

Jo-Von Tucker

In 1989 at age fifty-two, Jo-Von Tucker's life as she knew it came to a screeching halt. She was diagnosed with COPD and told she would be dependent on oxygen twenty-four hours a day for the rest of her life and had only two to five years to live.

Determined to beat the odds, Jo-Von set out to learn all she could about COPD, but found little. As a result she made it her mission to do all she could to provide information and support to people with COPD, and their families.

Prior to her COPD diagnosis Jo-Von owned a successful direct marketing consulting firm, JVT Direct Marketing, specializing in upscale catalogs. In the course of her career she received more than 400 national and international design, writing, and marketing awards. She was named one of the Top 20 U.S. Women Entrepreneurs in 1978 as well as 1978 Advertising Woman of the Year. She traveled extensively, speaking and consulting to those in the direct marketing industry.

After learning of her condition she moved to Cape Cod, Massachusetts, and acquired Clambake Celebrations, a company specializing in marketing and shipping live, fresh lobster clambake feasts throughout the United States. Clambake Celebrations was soon selected as one of the Top 100 Small Business Websites in America by *Small Business Computing Magazine.*

Jo-Von's enthusiasm and leadership in the COPD world made a positive change in the lives of many people. As founder and leader of the Cape Cod COPD Support Group she created a sense of sharing and community for people with the disease. Her newsletters, distributed to patients and health care professionals throughout the country, contained articles of current events in the world of COPD, locally and nationally. In a personal editorial each month she offered insight and information into life with COPD, often revealing her hopes, aspirations and fears. These editorials were, for many, the first and most often read feature of each newsletter.

Ms. Tucker was active in a number of efforts advocating for COPD awareness and patient empowerment. When attending COPD events she could always be counted on to not only see things through the patient's eyes but to speak out on their behalf. She was a fighter.

Her words had impact. When Jo-Von talked, everyone listened.

Jo-Von is the author of *Courage and Information for Life with COPD*, a groundbreaking work combining scientific and medical information about COPD with a patient's unique insights. She also published *Perspectives*, a book of her own poetry and photography. Born in Dallas, Texas, she attended the University of Texas in Austin, and lived and worked in New York for many years before moving to Cape Cod. Ms. Tucker passed away unexpectedly in late 2003 from complications following surgery. Her work, and her words, will continue to influence patients and compel them to take an active role in their care.

Additional Contributors

Robert A. Sandhaus, MD, PhD, FCCP

Dr. Sandhaus has nearly forty years of experience in medicine and research aimed at improving understanding Alpha1-antitrypsin deficiency and related disorders. He is board-certified in the specialty areas of internal medicine, pulmonary disease, and critical care medicine.

A principal investigator for the NIH Alpha1-Antitrypsin Deficiency Registry in the early 1990s, Dr. Sandhaus is a founding member of the Boards of Directors of AlphaNet and the Alpha-1 Foundation. He joined the biopharmaceutical industry in 1994 and helped lead the clinical departments of Cortech, Inc., NeXstar Pharmaceuticals, and Gilead Sciences over the subsequent six years, before accepting a position with AlphaNet and the Alpha-1 Foundation in April of 2000. He is now Clinical Director of the Alpha-1 Foundation, and Medical Director and Executive Vice President of AlphaNet.

Since 1981 Dr. Sandhaus has been a faculty member at National Jewish Health in Denver, Colorado, caring for one of the largest, continuously-followed groups of individuals with Alpha-1 in the world. He currently serves as Professor of Medicine and Director of the Alpha-1 Program at National Jewish Health.

With a B.A. in Molecular Biology from Haverford College, Dr. Sandhaus went on to receive a PhD in experimental pathology and a medical degree at Stony Brook University. He has held academic positions at Harvard Medical School, the University of California at San Francisco, and the University of Colorado. Dr. Sandhaus was born in Cleveland, Ohio. He now lives in Bow Mar, Colorado, with his family.

Francis V. Adams, MD

Dr. Adams is a pulmonologist in private practice in New York City, an Assistant Professor of Clinical Medicine at New York University, and an Attending Physician at the NYU Langone Medical Center and Bellevue Hospital in New York.

In 2006 Dr. Adams was sworn in as a police surgeon for the NYPD. He is the author of *The Asthma Sourcebook* (McGraw Hill) which is now in the 3rd Edition, *The Breathing Disorders Sourcebook* (McGraw Hill), and *Healing Through Empathy* (iUniverse). Dr. Adams is a contributor to *The LA Times* and hosts the weekly *Doctor Radio* show on Sirius/XM satellite radio. He has been named as one of the best doctors in the city by *New York Magazine* and in *Top Doctors: New York Metro Area* by Castle Connolly Medical Ltd.

Dr. Adams has been interviewed on television, radio, and the Internet in regard to his books, and has been quoted on the subject of asthma in newspaper and magazine articles. He has maintained a web site (www.adamsmd.com) for several years, which includes a News page that lists the current advances in lung disease. Dr. Adams publishes an electronic newsletter weekly, which is obtainable through his web site.

Dr. Adams received his BA from Georgetown University and his medical degree from Cornell Medical College.

Vijai Sharma, PhD

In 1994 Vijai Sharma, a clinical psychologist with over 30 years experience, was diagnosed with emphysema after suffering with untreated asthma and chronic bronchitis since childhood. In addition to a program of wide-ranging exercise, nutrition and self-care, he strictly follows the recommended COPD medical treatment.

Dr. Sharma specializes in mind-body medicine and appreciates how anxiety, depression, anger, pain, and stress, can affect cardiopulmonary, colon, and immune system function. He believes we can utilize the body, breath, mind, and spiritual energy, for personal well being, overall health, and a better quality of life.

Dr. Sharma received extensive clinical training in India, the United Kingdom, and Sweden, and has been licensed as a clinical psychologist in Tennessee since 1981. As a certified yoga teacher he has been registered with US Yoga Alliance (500+hours) since 2004 and has completed advance teachers' training in Yoga. Since being diagnosed he believes yoga has helped him psychologically and physically in his battle with emphysema.

Dr. Sharma has developed two exercise DVDs and companion workbooks, "Stretching and Breathing Exercises for Severe COPD," and "Stretching and Breathing for COPD." His clinical focus is on developing psychosocial interventions for anxiety and depression in COPD, and he presents nationally on Cognitive Behavioral Therapy and Yoga Breathing Techniques specifically for people with COPD. He has written over three hundred self-care articles for people and their families struggling with chronic illnesses. For specific COPD information: www.mindpub. com and http://www.mindpub.com/copdhome.htm.

Helen Sorenson, MA, RRT, CPFT, FAARC

Helen Sorenson is a registered respiratory therapist, and an Associate Professor in the Department of Respiratory Care at the University of Texas Health Science Center in San Antonio, Texas.

She received a degree in Biology from Dana College in Blair, Nebraska; a Certificate of Completion from California College for Respiratory Care and earned the CRT, RRT, and CPFT credentials from The National Board for Respiratory Care. In 2000 she was awarded a Master of Arts (MA) in Social Gerontology from the University of Nebraska, in Omaha, Nebraska. Mrs. Sorenson's passion for the art of respiratory care and helping patients breathe better is evident in everything she does.

In addition to the joy of her three children and five grandchildren, Mrs. Sorenson enjoys writing, playing the guitar, and reading. She is a published author currently at work on a second geriatric care textbook.

Resources

Alpha-1 Advocacy Alliance
http://www.alpha1advocacy.org
866-367-2122

The Alpha-1 Association
http://www.alpha1.org
800-521-3025

Alpha-1 confidential research registry
www.alphaoneregistry.org
877-886-2383

Alpha-One Foundation
www.alphaone.org
877-228-7321

Alpha-1 Genetic Counseling Center
Confidential genetic counseling for individuals in the Alpha-1 community. An expert resource for healthcare professionals.
http://www.alpha1.org
800-785-3177

American Association of Cardiovascular and Pulmonary Rehabilitation (AACVPR)
http://www.aacvpr.org
312-321-5146

American Lung Association
http://www.lungusa.org
800-586-4872

American Sleep Apnea Association
http://www.sleepapnea.org/
202-293-3650

Breathing Better, Living Well - Online information and support http://www.breathing-betterlivingwell.com
http://www.copdsupport.com
PO Box 2043
Holland, MI 49423

But You Don't Look Sick - Information and support for chronic disease, The Spoon Theory
http://www.butyoudontlooksick.com

COPD Canada
http://www.copdcanada.ca/

The COPD Digest
http://www.copddigest.org
866-316-2673

The COPD Foundation
http://www.copdfoundation.org
866-731-2673

COPD Information Line
866-316-2673

COPD International – Online information and support
http://COPD-International.com

COPD Support, INC. – Online information and support
http://COPD-Support1.com

COPDsurvivors – Online information and support
http://health.groups.yahoo.com/group/COPDsurvivors/

EFFORTS (Emphysema Foundation for our right to Survive) - Online information and support
www.emphysema.net

Health Central COPD Connection
http://www.healthcentral.com/copd/

Learn More, Breathe Better Campaign – Promoting awareness and education of COPD
http://www.nhlbi.nih.gov/health/public/lung/copd/lmbb-campaign/index.htm

Love your Lungs – Information and support
http://www.loveyourlungs-breatheforlife.com/

Mind Publications – Information about relaxation, yoga, stress, anxiety and depression in COPD
http://www.mindpub.com

National Heart, Lung and Blood Institute
http://nhlbi.nih.gov
301-592-8573

National Home Oxygen Patients Association
http://www.homeoxygen.org

National Jewish Health – Top respiratory hospital
http://www.nationaljewish.org
800-222-5864

National Lung Health Education Program
http://www.nhlep.org

Portable Oxygen
http://www.portableoxygen.org

Pulmonary Education and Research Foundation (PERF)
http://www.perf2ndwind.org
310-539-8390

The Pulmonary Paper
http://www.pulmonarypaper.org
800-950-3698

Sea Puffers – Pulmonary Cruises
http://www.seapuffers.com
866-673-3019

Second wind Lung Transplant Association, Inc.
http://www.2ndwind.org
888-855-9463

US COPD Coalition
http://uscopdcoalition.org
877-341-2673

Your Lung Health
http://www.yourlunghealth.org
972-243-227

Well Spouse Foundation – for family members and other caregivers
http://www.wellspouse.org
800-838-0879

Illustration – The Lungs

The Lungs

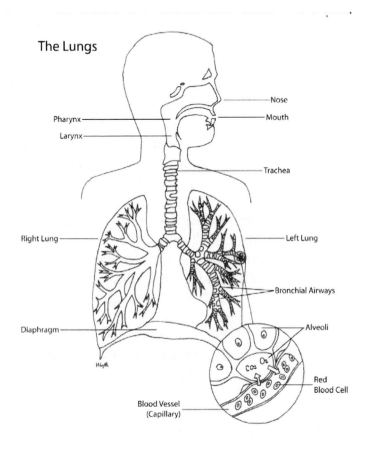

Glossary

Acute: An illness that comes on suddenly and lasts a few hours or days.

Airway Obstruction: A blocking or narrowing of the airways on their way to or within the lung.

Allergen: A substance causing inflammation in the lungs. Common allergens are pollen, animal dander, dust mites and mold.

Alpha-1 Antitrypsin Deficiency: A genetically inherited condition in which the liver does not make enough of a protein that protects the lungs and liver from damage, leading to emphysema and liver disease. Patients with Alpha-1 Antitrypsin Deficiency develop severe emphysema in their 20's, 30's or 40's.

Alveoli: Tiny, sac-like structures at the ends of the airways where oxygen and carbon dioxide exchange takes place.

Antibiotic: A drug that kills or inhibits bacteria.

Apnea: The absence of breathing, usually longer than 10 seconds. Obstructive sleep apnea is a condition in which breathing stops during sleep due to an obstruction in the airway. Central sleep apnea is a condition in which, for some reason, the respiratory center in the brain fails to send the message to breathe.

Arterial Blood Gas (ABG): A blood test drawn from the artery to determine how well the lungs are working relative to other metabolic functions of the body.

Asthma: An obstructive lung disease characterized by airway hyper-responsiveness, inflammation, narrowing and spasm.

Asthmatic Bronchitis: A type of bronchitis commonly associated with COPD involving cough, airway hyper-responsiveness, and mucous production.

Bacteria: Infectious organisms that may produce bronchitis or pneumonia as well as illness elsewhere in the body.

BiPAP (Bi-level Positive Airway Pressure - inspiratory and expiratory): A mechanical device used to assist breathing in severe lung disease, following surgery, or in obstructive sleep apnea. This treatment is "non-invasive", meaning that no tube is inserted into the lungs. Pressure is applied to the respiratory airways via a mask that can be quite easily and quickly put on and removed.

Bleb: Destroyed, non-functional part of the lung that takes up space and puts pressure on a less damaged portion of the lung.

Bronchial Hygiene: Keeping the lungs free of excess mucous by using inhalers, nebulizer treatments, percussion and postural drainage, systemic hydration, effective cough techniques or mechanical devices that aid in airway clearance.

Bronchitis: Irritation of the lining of the bronchial tubes, characterized by a frequent cough.

Bronchiectasis: Chronic infection often found in the lower parts of the lung, characterized by copious amounts of excess mucous.

Bronchus: The two main divisions from the trachea, each one leading into a lung. There are approximately twenty additional sets of branches before reaching the alveoli, where oxygen and carbon dioxide exchange take place.

Cannula (pronounced: Can′-yoo-luh): A soft plastic device used to deliver oxygen. Worn on the face and held in place by the ears, it has two short prongs positioned in the nares.

Capillaries: Tiny blood vessels surrounding the alveoli through which oxygen and carbon dioxide pass on the way into and out of the lungs.

Carbon Dioxide (CO_2): The waste product of respiration that is removed from the body through exhalation.

Chronic: Disease that has been present for a longer period of time, usually months or years.

Cilia: Tiny, hair like structures that line the bronchial airways and sweep mucous upward toward the mouth. Cilia are important to cleanse the lungs and defend against irritants, and can be destroyed by cigarette smoke and pollution.

Cor Pulmonale: Strain of the right side of the heart due to lung disease.

CPAP (Continuous Positive Airway Pressure - inspiratory): A mechanical device used to assist breathing and in the treatment of obstructive sleep apnea. This treatment is "non-invasive", meaning that no tube is inserted into the lungs. Pressure is applied to the respiratory airways via a mask that can be quite easily and quickly put on and removed.

Diaphragm: The main muscle of breathing. The diaphragm is a large sheet of muscle separating the chest and the abdomen.

Dyspnea: Difficulty breathing, shortness of breath.

Emphysema: Destruction or enlargement of the alveoli; a condition in which the alveoli lose their elasticity and become stretched out and floppy.

Exacerbation: An episodic worsening of a chronic illness.

FEV$_1$: Forced Expiratory Volume in the first second of exhalation in a Pulmonary Function Test. Is helpful in determining the degree of airway obstruction.

Holding chamber: A handheld device, usually plastic, containing a one-way valve, used with a metered dose inhaler (MDI) assisting in maximum delivery of medication to the lungs.

Inflammation: Irritated, reddened, and swollen tissue.

Irritants: Substances that irritate the airways, causing swelling and increased mucous production. Common irritants are smoke, smog, aerosol sprays, and perfume.

Metabolism: The consumption of nutrients combined with oxygen, which produces energy and maintains living tissue.

Nebulizer: A breathing treatment in which liquid medication becomes a fine mist to be inhaled into the lungs. Can be taken in a medical facility or at home.

Obstructive sleep apnea (OSA): A blockage of the airway causing the absence of breathing during sleep, sometimes hundreds of times during the night and often for a minute or longer.

Oxygen: (O_2): A gas needed in order to sustain human life. Earth's atmosphere is 20.9% oxygen.

Oxygen Saturation (O_2 Sat): A measure of the amount of oxygen in the blood, measured in percent and often obtained with a pulse oximeter.

Pneumonia: A common infection in people with COPD caused by bacteria or virus.

Pneumothorax: Lung collapse causing air to leak from within the lung into the space between the lung and the chest wall, causing pain and difficulty breathing.

Pulmonary Function Test: A medical test performed by a patient, resulting in measurements of air movement – speed, volume, and flow – as well as diffusion of oxygen. Can be done in a complete or abbreviated form depending upon information required by the physician.

Pulse Oximeter: A device used to determine the percent of oxygen saturation in the blood. This test is non-invasive (nothing is placed inside the body), painless, and quickly and easily done.

Pursed Lips Breathing: A method of breathing which prolongs the expiratory phase, increasing the amount of carbon dioxide expelled, slowing down breathing and allowing the person using this method to increase control over breathing.

Respiratory Failure: A chronic or acute state in which the lungs are unable to provide enough oxygen to the body and/or remove enough carbon dioxide from the body.

Sleep Study: A study done to observe various physiologic changes during sleep. Done overnight in a laboratory.

SOB: Short of Breath, or Shortness of Breath

Spacer: A handheld device, usually plastic, used with metered dose inhaler (MDI) assisting in increased delivery of medication to the lungs.

Spirometer: A device used to measure lung function.

Spirometry: A lung function test measuring the volume and speed of air being inhaled and exhaled.

Trachea: The main airway leading to both lungs. Sometimes referred to as the windpipe.

Transtracheal Catheter: A small tube inserted into a hole in the trachea supplying oxygen to the lungs. Used for long-term supplemental oxygen use in which a higher flow is required and / or if the patient does not wish to have a nasal cannula visible.

Ventilator: A mechanical device used to treat respiratory failure or provide respiratory support following surgery. Tubing from the ventilator is connected to an endotracheal tube inserted into the patient's lungs via the mouth or nose. Mechanical ventilation is considered to be an invasive treatment, meaning that something is inserted into the body. Also referred to as a respirator.

Virus: A group of highly contagious infectious agents causing head colds and chest infections, as well as illness elsewhere in the body. Antibiotics are ineffective against viruses. Vaccination against the influenza virus (flu shot) is effective.

Wheeze: A whistling sound of air entering or leaving the lungs. Can be a sign of muscle spasm around the airways, commonly found in asthma.

Early Warning Signs of Acute Exacerbation of COPD

* A change in your cough – are you coughing more, less, or is it different than usual?
* A change in the amount or color of your sputum. Is it yellow, green, or bloody? Your mucous should be clear or white.
* If you have a pulse oximeter at home, are your O2 sats (oxygen saturations) lower than usual?
* Sudden weight gain such as 3-5 lbs. overnight.
* Swelling in your ankles or feet. Here's a tip: Gently press the tip of your finger into the skin around your ankles and feet. Does it leave a dent? It shouldn't. If it does, call your doctor.
* Morning dizziness, confusion, or headache that doesn't go away with medications such as Tylenol or Advil.
* A heart rate faster than usual (60-100 is normal with each person having their own "normal"). Know your normal resting heart rate.
* Your urine should be pale yellow and clear, with no odor. If it is darker than usual, cloudy, or with a foul odor, you might have a urinary tract infection.
* Fever.
* Unusual fatigue.
* Joint or muscle aches.
* Other_____
  _____
  _____

(over)

My Exacerbation Prevention Plan:

_____

_____

_____

_____

_____

_____

Dr. _____

Office phone number: _____